Health Facilities

1995–96 Review

First published in the United States of America by:
Rockport Publishers, Inc.
146 Granite Street
Rockport, Massachusetts 01966-1299
Telephone 508 546 9590
Fax 508 546 7141

Other Distribution by:
Rockport Publishers
Rockport, Massachusetts 01966-1299

Distributed to the book trade and art trade by
The AIA Press
1735 New York Avenue
Washington, DC 20006
Telephone 800 365 2724
Fax 802 864 7626

ISBN 1-55835-140-X

10 9 8 7 6 5 4 3 2 1

1995 AIA Academy of Architecture for Health

Joseph G. Sprague, FAIA, *President*
Morris A. Stein, AIA, *President-Elect*
Janet Baum, AIA
Ronald B. Blitch, AIA
Georgeann B. Burns, Assoc. AIA
D. Kirk Hamilton, FAIA
Donald C. McKahan, AIA
Arthur N. Tuttle, Jr., AIA

1995 Jury

Ronald B. Blitch, AIA
Daniel M. Buxbaum, Ph.D.
Dr. Jules I. Levine
Barbara A. Nadel, AIA, Jury Chair
Gerald F. Oudens, AIA

AIA Staff, Health Facilities: 1995–96 Review

Elizabeth M. White, *Director*, AIA Academy of Architecture for Health
Jane C. Opera, *Information Coordinator*

ART DIRECTOR: Lynne Havighurst
DESIGN: Group C, Inc.
LAYOUT: Jennie Bush, Books By Design, Inc.
PAGING: Carol Keller
COVER PHOTOGRAPH: Lenscape, Inc. *(project appears on p. 151)*

Manufactured in Hong Kong by
Regent Publishing Services Limited

Health Facilities

1995–96

Review

The American Institute of Architects Press

Washington, D.C.

Contents

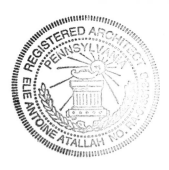

1995 Jury

BARBARA A. NADEL, AIA, jury chair, is principal of Barbara Nadel Architect, a New York City architectural firm specializing in programming, planning, and design of health care, institutional, and correctional facilities.

Ms. Nadel is chair of the design committee of the AIA Academy of Architecture for Health, a director on the New York State Board of Directors, and is chair of the AIA New York Chapter Health Facilities Committee. She was the AIA New York State delegate to the White House briefing with Vice President Gore on Health Care Reform and Small Business.

Ms. Nadel's articles have appeared in numerous national publications, including Architectural Record, Progressive Architecture, American City & County, Texas Architect, Home Office Computing, Corrections Today, Sheriff, and American Airlines' Latitudes South.

RONALD B. BLITCH, AIA, is president of Blitch Architects, Inc. in New Orleans, specializing in the design of health care facilities and retirement communities in the Gulf South. He has won more than 30 national, regional, and local awards for design excellence, including the 1994 Award for Critical Care Design from AIA, the Society of Critical Care Medicine, and the American Association of Critical Care Nurses. He has served as president of AIA Louisiana, and currently is vice president of the AIA's Academy of Architecture for Health, a charter board member of the AIA's Aging Design Research Program, and host chapter chair for the 1997 AIA national convention in New Orleans.

DANIEL M. BUXBAUM, Ph.D., is director of space and facilities planning at Vanderbilt University Medical Center. Over the past twenty years he has been involved in the programming, planning, design, and construction of a new medical campus which includes three hospitals, an ambulatory care center, a wellness center, two medical office facilities, three biomedical research facilities and a biomedical library. Over the past ten years, he has managed an average of nearly 100 renovation projects per year.

JULES I. LEVINE, Ph.D., received a bachelor's degree in electrical engineering from the University of Virginia, a master's degree in management sciences and operations research from Johns Hopkins University, and a Ph.D. in biomedical engineering from the University of Virginia. He has been on the faculty at the University of Virginia since 1972 and directed the Center for Delivery of Health Care.

He has served as associate dean of the School of Medicine, and currently as associate vice president for health sciences, and is responsible for all planning and facilities development for the Health Sciences Center. Dr. Levine recently served as project director for the $230 million replacement hospital project at the University of Virginia. His current responsibilities include planning and development of research, ambulatory care, and inpatient facilities, as well as strategic and general planning for the Health Sciences Center.

GERALD F. OUDENS, AIA, a founding principal of Oudens + Knoop, Architects, PC, Washington, D.C., has been responsible for the programming and design of hospital and health care projects located in diverse parts of the United States and in Central America, Africa, Europe, and the Middle East. He is past president of the AIA Academy of Architecture for Health and has been active in teaching, research, speaking, and publishing on health care design issues. He has participated in numerous advisory panels and design juries. Among his firm's many awards are two design citations in previous issues of the AIA's Health Facilities Review.

Jury Statement

The 102 submissions to the 1995–96 Health Facilities Review represented a broad spectrum of project types from all parts of the country. There were many ambulatory care facilities and fewer major large hospital and academic medical center projects than in the past.

The jury found excellence in a variety of projects. For example, a 6,900-square-foot neighborhood primary care center achieved multiple objectives within limited resources and difficult building and site constraints. In contrast, an unbuilt 450,000-square-foot medical complex promises excellence without such stringent design or budget limitations.

The jury noted that many of the submitted projects paid more attention to public spaces than patient service areas. In some of the larger hospital projects, a number of "strange bedfellows" or unusual adjacencies were observed.

Many projects, while competently executed, were deemed to be without any unique or compelling design response to the program or the built environment. The jury saw numerous examples of traditional, formulaic design approaches that were often inconsistent with the architect's statements. While many architect's statements acknowledged the emerging concerns of health care delivery, the projects did not always reflect these issues. The jury expects that future submissions will address the impact of changes in health care delivery and that new approaches will emerge as demands evolve.

Since this is the first Review to be published in color, legible floor plans and quality photography became particularly important factors for inclusion in the book. The jury also noted that some good projects were omitted because the graphics lacked both quality and clarity.

The jury for the 1995–96 Health Facilities Review included three health care architects and planners and two senior health care administrators. Over the course of the two-day process, the jury discussed and debated the merits of each project. Final decisions for citations and inclusions were unanimous in all cases.

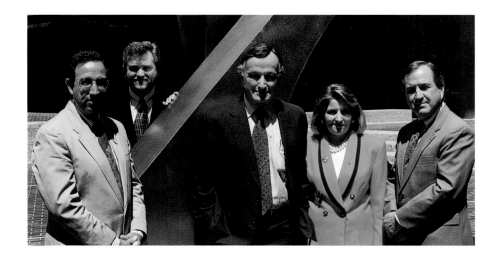

Left to right: Daniel Buxbaum, Ph.D.;
Ronald Blitch, AIA;
Gerald Oudens, AIA;
Barbara Nadel, AIA, jury chair;
Jules Levine, Ph.D.

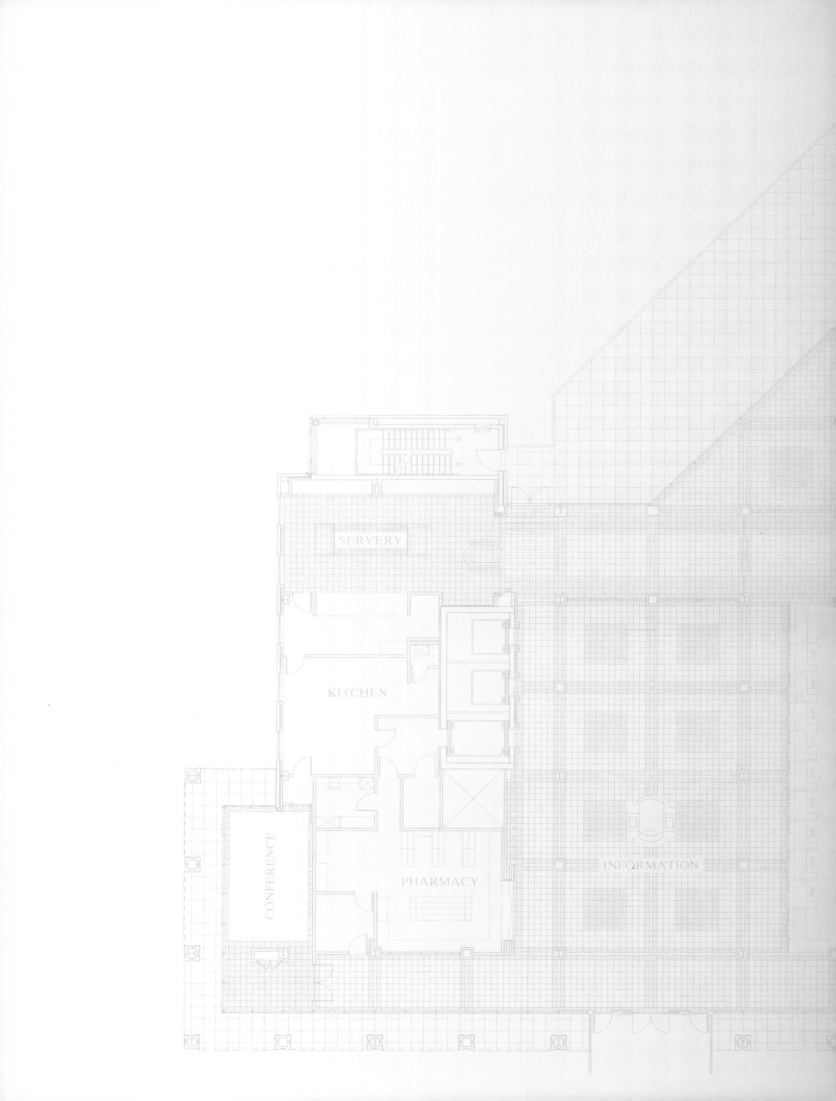

Ambulatory Care Centers

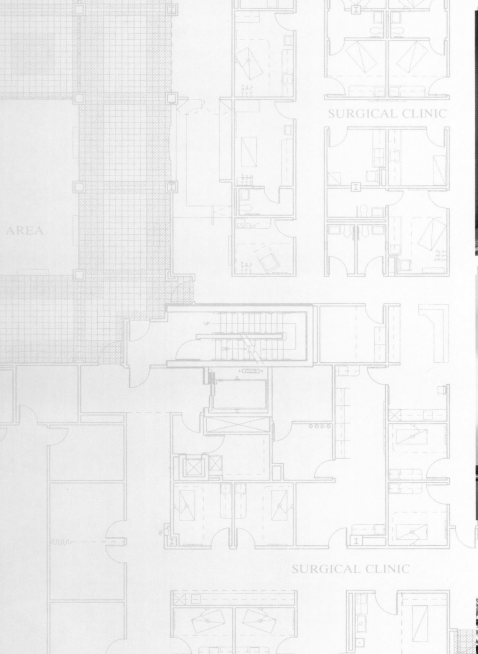

SURGICAL CLINIC

WAITING AREA

SURGICAL CLINIC

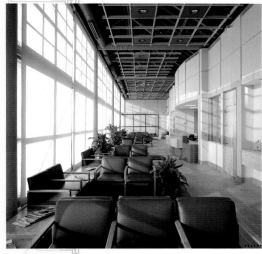

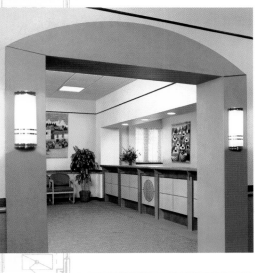

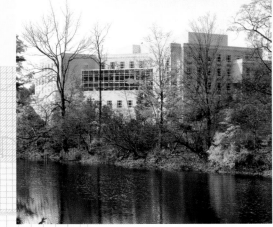

The Carl J. Shapiro Clinical Center, Beth Israel HealthCare

Boston, Massachusetts

Citation

This major project on a congested urban site in Boston successfully defers to and integrates the smaller-scale 1929 Massachusetts College of Art on the site. The stepped massing of the ambulatory care building and its use of forms and materials allow both structures to coexist comfortably. The project was most successful in this blending of old and new. The typical functions of the ambulatory care floor are well coordinated with the facade treatments. Patient circulation and orientation are clear and straightforward, and the flow between floors and functions is evident and rational. The atrium space between the old and the new is an effective bridge between the two structures.

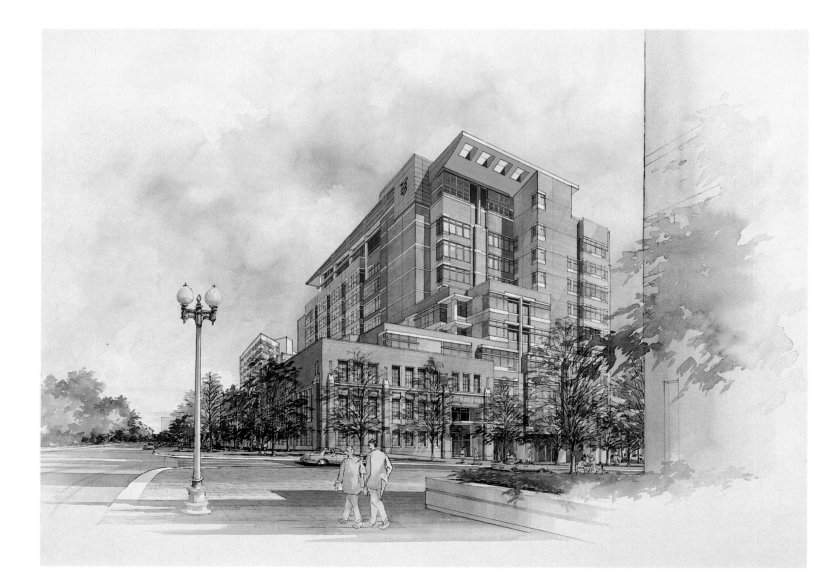

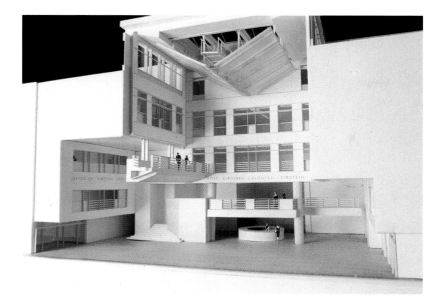

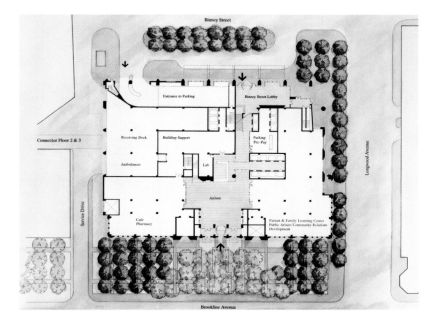

ARCHITECT'S STATEMENT

In creating a modern, ambulatory care facility on the site of a historic structure that was to be partially preserved, the design team confronted an elementary question: whether to imitate, deny, or integrate the existing architecture. Integration—the most challenging option and the one holding the greatest potential rewards—was the avenue chosen. A major design challenge for the new clinical center was to integrate the larger mass of the new building with the preserved portions of the historic structure without making the facade appear as a minor historic appendage. In keeping with the aim of expanding on the historic structure's existing design elements, the exterior of the new building incorporates materials, colors, texture, and scaling devices that are contemporary yet relate to the brickwork, detail, ornament, and mass of the original

site. The integration philosophy was carried into the interior public spaces, where a four-story atrium was created to link the old and new structures. The atrium serves not only as a functional link, but also reinvigorates the facade of the historic college building by incorporating it within the new building.

Owner
Beth Israel Hospital

Data

Type of Facility
Ambulatory care building

Context
Hospital-based

Type of Construction
New

Area of Building
690,500 GSF (including five levels of parking)

Cost of Construction
Bid estimate: $88,500,000

Cost of Medical Equipment
Bid estimate: $23,600,000

Status of Project
Estimated completion date: December 1995

Credits

Client Representatives
Mitchell T. Rabkin, M.D., President

Francis J. Sullivan, V.P. Facilities Planning & Engineering

Robert Flack, Project Manager

Architect
Rothman Rothman Heineman Architects Inc.
711 Atlantic Avenue
Boston, Massachusetts 02111

Consulting Architects
Chan Krieger & Associates, Inc.
1132 Massachusetts Avenue
Cambridge, Massachusetts 02138

Solomon + Bauer Architects, Inc.
44 Hunt Street
Watertown, Massachusetts 02172

Consulting Interior Designer
Lloy Hack Associates, Inc.
Boston, Massachusetts

Landscape Architect
Child Associates, Inc.
Boston, Massachusetts

Structural Engineer
LeMessurier Consultants
Cambridge, Massachusetts

(credits continue)

Credits (continued)

Mechanical Engineer

BR+A Consulting Engineers, Inc.
Boston, Massachusetts

Electrical Engineer

Lottero + Mason Associates, Inc.
Boston, Massachusetts

Plumbing and Fire Protection Engineer

Robert W. Sullivan, Inc.
Boston, Massachusetts

Civil Engineer

Vanasse Hangen Brustlin, Inc.
Watertown, Massachusetts

Geotechnical Engineer

Haley & Aldrich
Cambridge, Massachusetts

Lead Subgrade Engineer

Parsons Brinckerhoff Quade
& Douglas
Boston, Massachusetts

Contractors

Macomber Construction
(exterior shell/core and sitework)
Boston, Massachusetts

Kiewit Eastern Co.
(below-grade garage)
Southborough, Massachusetts

Beacon Construction Company
(interior fit-out)
Boston, Massachusetts

Photographers

David Desroches
(building models)
Boston, Massachusetts

R. Alan Lewis and Tom Sieniewicz
(atrium model)
Rothman Rothman Heineman
Architects Inc./Chan Krieger
& Associates Inc.

Renderings

Dongik Lee
Boston, Massachusetts

Martha Moncier
Rothman Rothman Heineman
Architects Inc.
Boston, Massachusetts

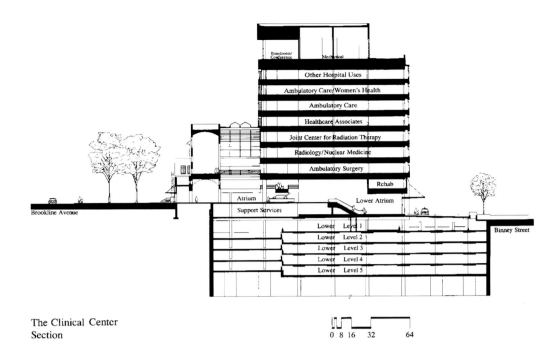

The Clinical Center
Section

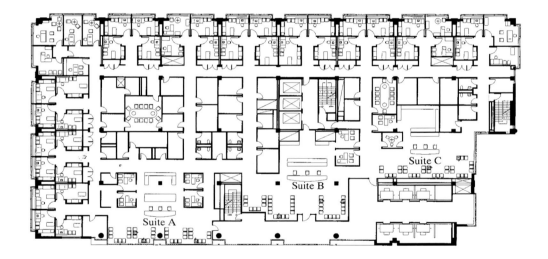

The Clinical Center
Ambulatory Care
Typical Upper Floor

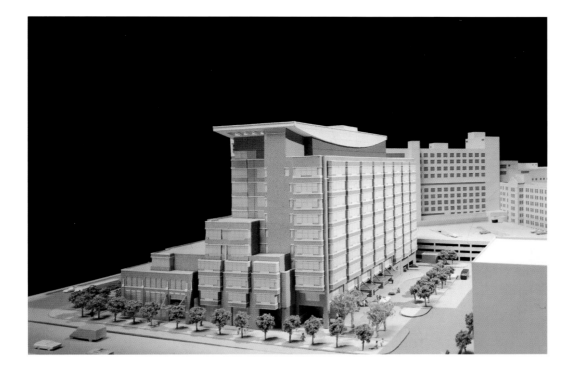

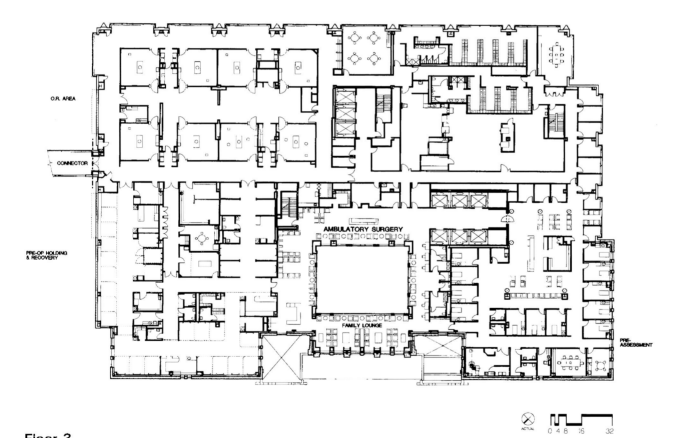

O.R. AREA

CONNECTOR

PRE-OP HOLDING
& RECOVERY

AMBULATORY SURGERY

FAMILY LOUNGE

PRE-
ASSESSMENT

ACTUAL 0 4 8 16 32

Floor 3

Alliance Surgery Center

Mount Holly, New Jersey

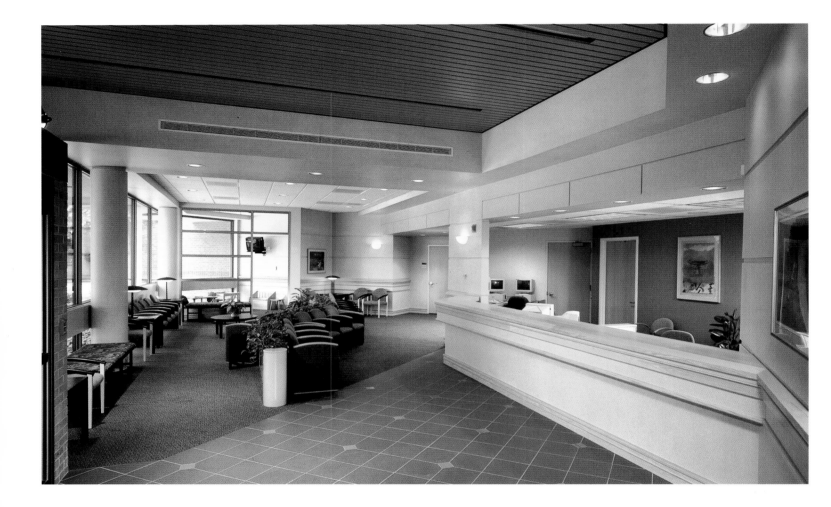

ARCHITECT'S STATEMENT

Located adjacent to the main hospital, this center replaces and expands the outpatient surgery program of the institution. The design uses natural light generously and makes a conscious attempt to create a friendly, therapeutic environment. Even the surgical core is flooded with light from a skylight that extends the length of its corridor.

The center is site-oriented so that its entrance aligns with and is visible from the main entrance of the hospital. This relationship is intended to create a visual bond between the two facilities and to impart a feeling of safety to its patients.

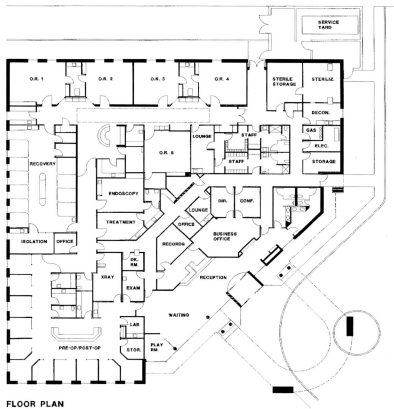

FLOOR PLAN

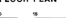

0   15   30

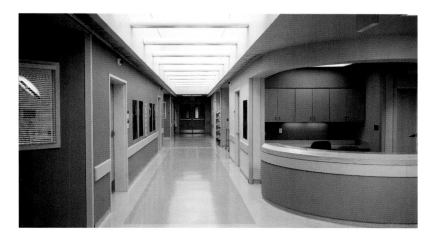

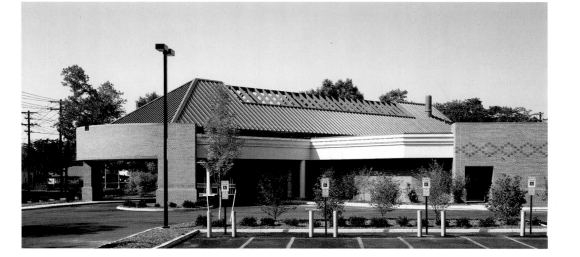

O w n e r
Memorial Health Alliance

D a t a

Type of Facility
Ambulatory surgery center

Context
Freestanding

Type of Construction
New

Area of Building
18,075 GSF

Cost of Construction
$4,257,900

Cost of Medical Equipment
$1,059,000

Status of Project
Completed January 1994

C r e d i t s

Architect
Costanza Spector Clauser
Architects
304 Harper Drive, Suite 100
Moorestown, New Jersey 08057

Structural Engineer
O'Donnell & Naccarato
Philadelphia, Pennsylvania

Mechanical/Electrical Engineer
Syska & Hennessy
Princeton, New Jersey

Medical Equipment Consultant
Help International
Plano, Texas

Furnishings and Accessories
Wendy Holden Associates
Moorestown, New Jersey

Contractor
R. M. Shoemaker
West Conshohocken, Pennsylvania

Photographer
Thomas Bernard
Berwyn, Pennsylvania

Ambulatory Center, Harris Methodist HEB

Bedford, Texas

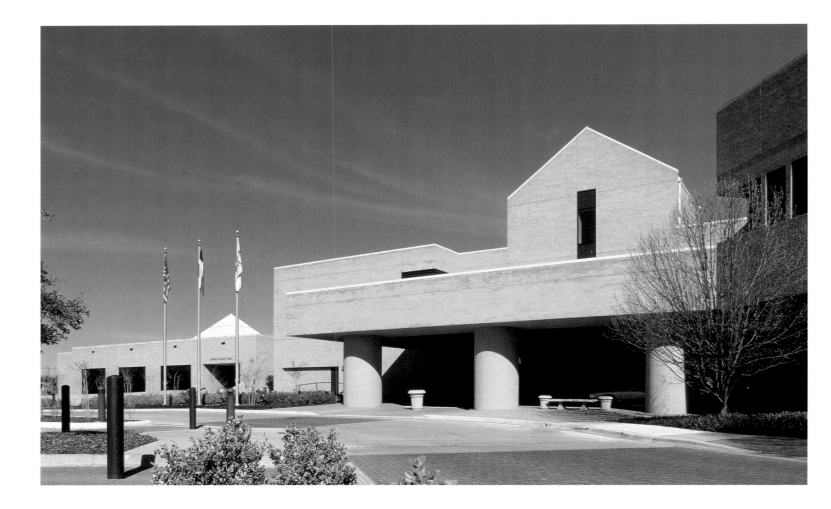

The object was to design an ambulatory center to support the outpatient load of the hospital and connect it to an existing cancer center. The design solution ties the hospital's main lobby to the cancer center by means of the upper-level mall. This skylighted mall is adjacent to an expanded porte cochere, which is, in effect, the medical center's front door.

The finishes in the mall are marble flooring, painted walls, and skylighted ceilings. The original lobby and the new mall with their richly lit, but never luxurious, spaces are now the heart of public circulation for this major suburban medical center.

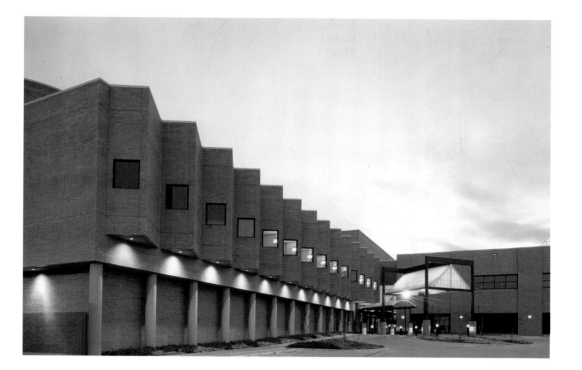

Owner
Harris Healthcare System

Data

Type of Facility
Ambulatory center

Context
Hospital-based: 30 beds

Type of Construction
New and renovation

Area of Building
88,694 GSF (69,163 new;
19,531 renovation)

Cost of Construction
$8,324,924
($6,916,300 new;
$1,426,624 renovation)

Cost of Medical Equipment
$1,433,888

Status of Project
Completed September 1993

Credits

Architect
Page Southerland Page
3500 Maple Avenue, Suite 700
Dallas, Texas 75219

Structural/Mechanical/Electrical Engineer
Page Southerland Page
Dallas, Texas

Contractor
HCB Contractors
Dallas, Texas

Photographer
Craig Blackmon, AIA, ASMP

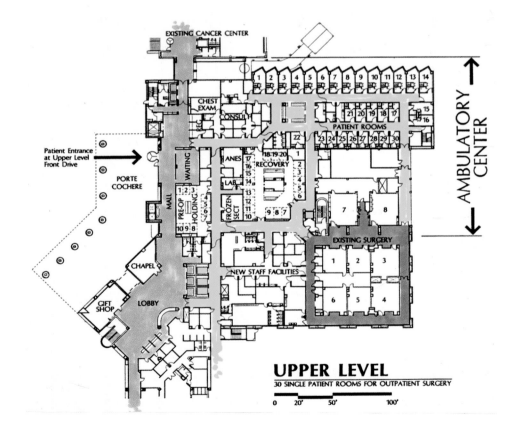

UPPER LEVEL
30 SINGLE PATIENT ROOMS FOR OUTPATIENT SURGERY

0   20'   50'   100'

The Mary Imogene Bassett Hospital: Bassett Clinic

Cooperstown, New York

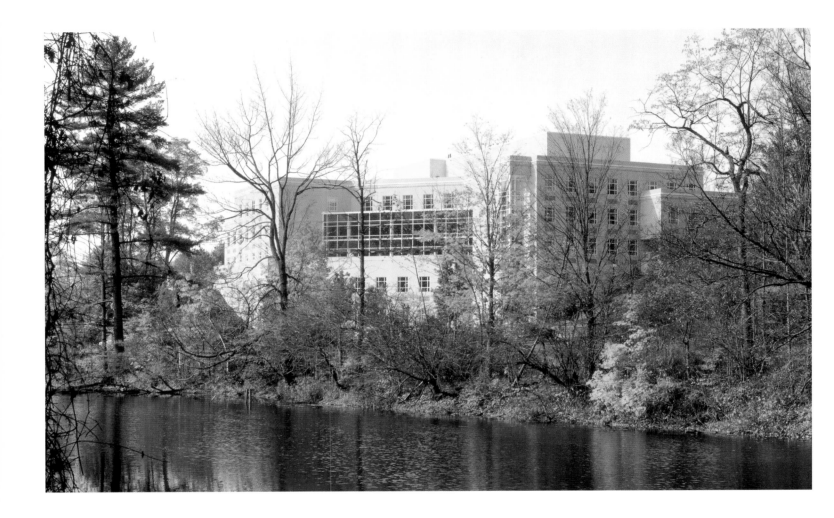

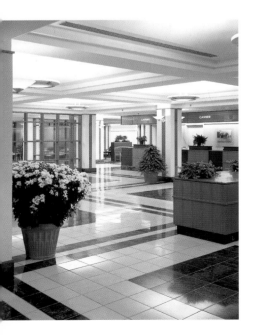

ARCHITECT'S STATEMENT

Bassett Clinic, located on a site overlooking the Susquehanna River, capitalizes on hillside topography to comply with the guidelines of the surrounding national historic district. Two stories are built into the hillside, with three terraced levels above grade. From the street, the building blends into the hospital campus and residential neighborhood. Viewed from the river, the structure appears to nestle into the embankment.

A central common space functions as the building's principal organizing element. Clinics wrap around two sides of the largely triangular building, with common areas on the remaining leg. Featuring views across the river, these public areas serve as an orientation point for both patients and visitors. A modular design concept ensures flexibility in meeting changes in service demand and anticipated growth.

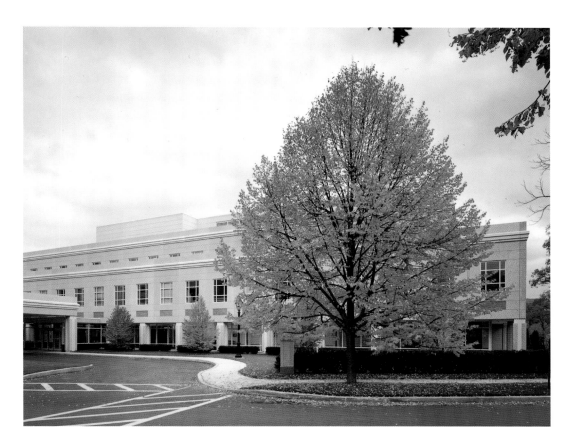

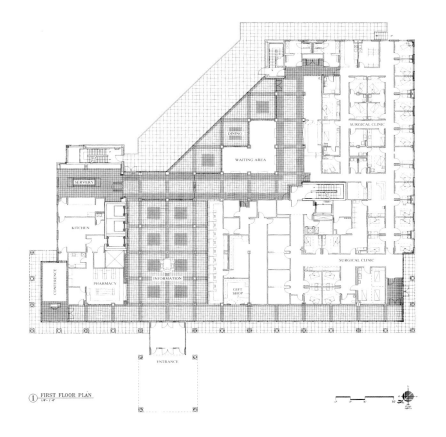

① FIRST FLOOR PLAN

Beth Israel Hospital and Children's Hospital Medical Care Center

Lexington, Massachusetts

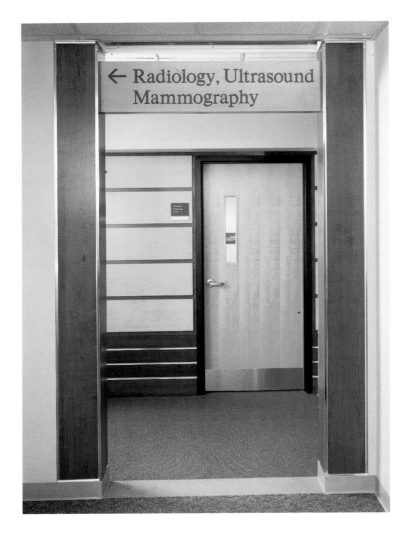

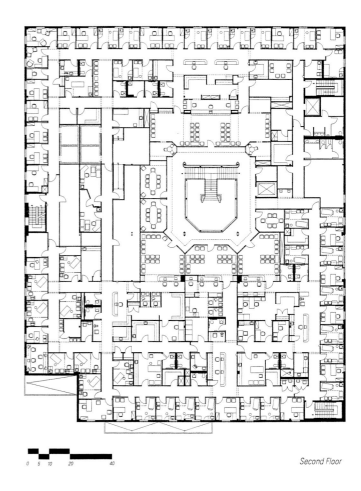

Second Floor

0   5   10   20   40

ARCHITECT'S STATEMENT

A two-story building previously used for manufacturing and corporate offices was renovated to include a state-of-the-art ambulatory health-care center. The building includes an ambulatory surgery suite with four operatories, a radiology suite, laboratory, physical and infusion therapy, primary care, and specialty services departments. The project was the collaborative effort of two hospitals that wanted to provide convenient and easy access to urban-quality academic medicine in a suburban setting. The center also provides diagnostic screening services to patients who otherwise would not receive them.

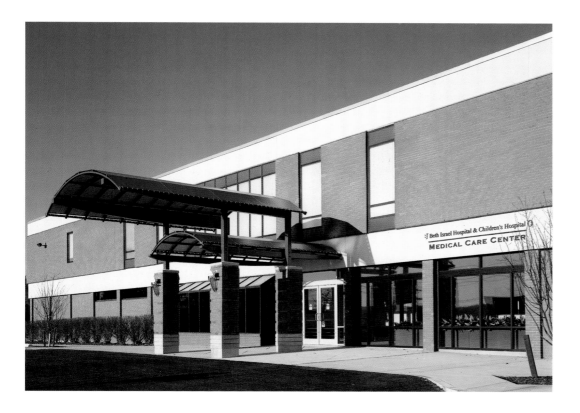

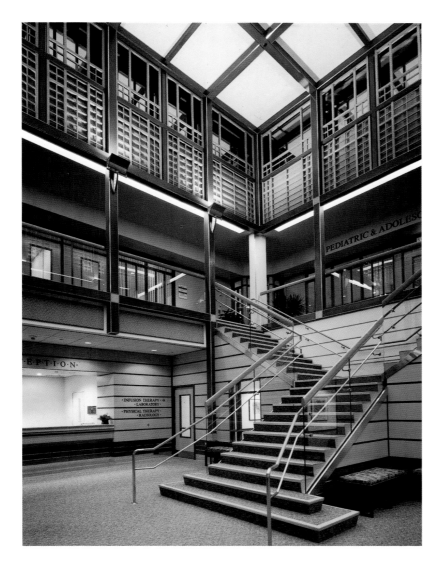

Owner
Beth Israel Hospital and Children's Hospital Joint Venture

Data

Type of Facility
Ambulatory health-care center

Context
Freestanding

Type of Construction
Renovation

Area of Building
57,924 GSF

Cost of Construction
$5,498,000

Cost of Medical Equipment
$2,900,000

Status of Project
Completed October 15, 1993

Credits

Architect
SBA | Steffian Bradley Associates, Inc.
100 North Washington
Boston, Massachusetts 02114

Structural Engineer
Charles Chaloff Consulting Engineers
Boston, Massachusetts

Mechanical Engineer
TMP Consulting Engineers, Inc.
Boston, Massachusetts

Electrical Engineer
Lottero + Mason Associates, Inc.
Boston, Massachusetts

Contractor
Kennedy & Ross
Arlington, Massachusetts

Photographers
Wayne Soverns, Jr.
Dorcester, Massachusetts

Brad Hutchins
Watertown, Massachusetts

Douglas Gilbert
Newburyport, Massachusetts

Beth Israel Medical Center

New York, New York

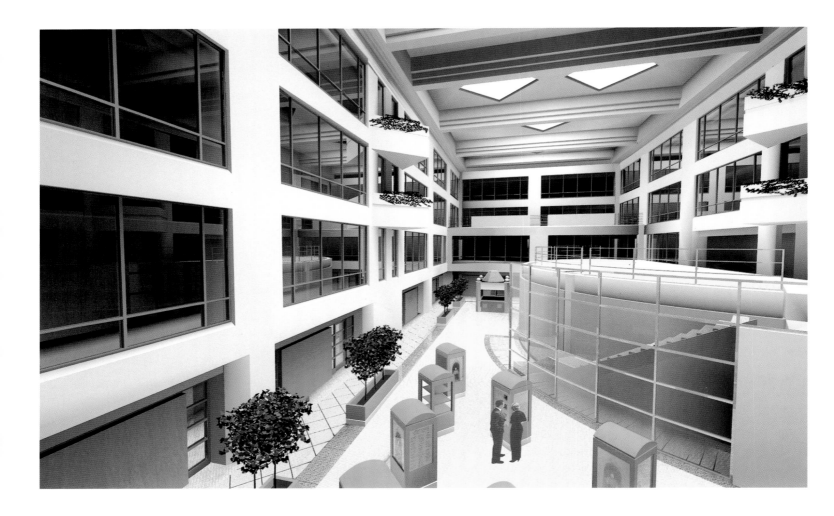

ARCHITECT'S STATEMENT

The Medical Center, a prestigious 974-bed teaching hospital in New York City, is moving all of its ambulatory care services into 300,000 square feet of space it purchased in a modern, mixed-use building several blocks from its main campus. Creative, adaptive re-use of this space includes: four-story, glass-enclosed atrium with auditorium; a series of intimate waiting areas that lead to a vast network of treatment rooms and labs; a "hidden" service corridor that circles each floor; "wet walls" between suites, but partition walls between offices to allow for flexible planning for the future; and patient records and x-ray rooms completely digitized in data banks with no hard copy.

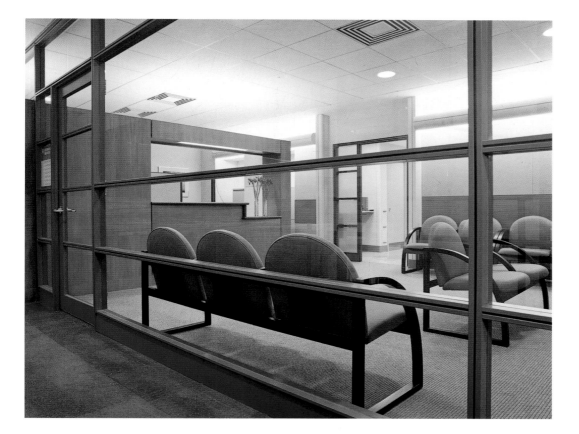

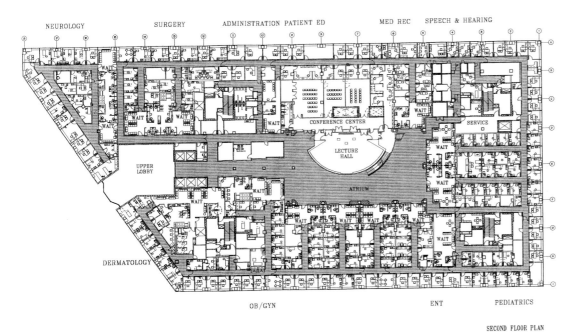

NEUROLOGY   SURGERY   ADMINISTRATION   PATIENT ED   MED REC   SPEECH & HEARING

CONFERENCE CENTER

SERVICE

WAIT

UPPER
LOBBY

WAIT

LECTURE
HALL

WAIT

ATRIUM

WAIT

WAIT

WAIT

WAIT

WAIT

DERMATOLOGY

OB/GYN   ENT   PEDIATRICS

SECOND FLOOR PLAN

SCALE

1'   10' 20'   40'   80'

Owner
Beth Israel Medical Center

Data
Type of Facility
Ambulatory care

Context
Freestanding

Type of Construction
Renovation

Area of Building
230,000 GSF

Cost of Construction
Bid estimate: $25,000,000

Cost of Medical Equipment
Bid estimate: $20,000,000

Status of Project
Estimated completion date:
January 1996

Credits
Architect
Larsen Associates/Architects
170 Varick Street
New York, New York 10013

Client Representative
Angelo Fanelli, P.E.
Vice President, Facilities
Management

Structural Engineer
Rosenwasser Grossman
New York, New York

Mechanical/Electrical Engineer
Cosentini Associates
New York, New York

Elevator Consultant
Calvin L. Kort
Glen Rock, New Jersey

Acoustical Consultant
Cerami & Associates
New York, New York

Audio/Visual Consultant
Gene Perlowin Associates, Inc.
New York, New York

Contractor
Lehrer McGovern Bovis
New York, New York

Photographer
Elliott Kaufman
New York, New York

Division of Cardiothoracic Surgery, Columbia Presbyterian Medical Center

New York, New York

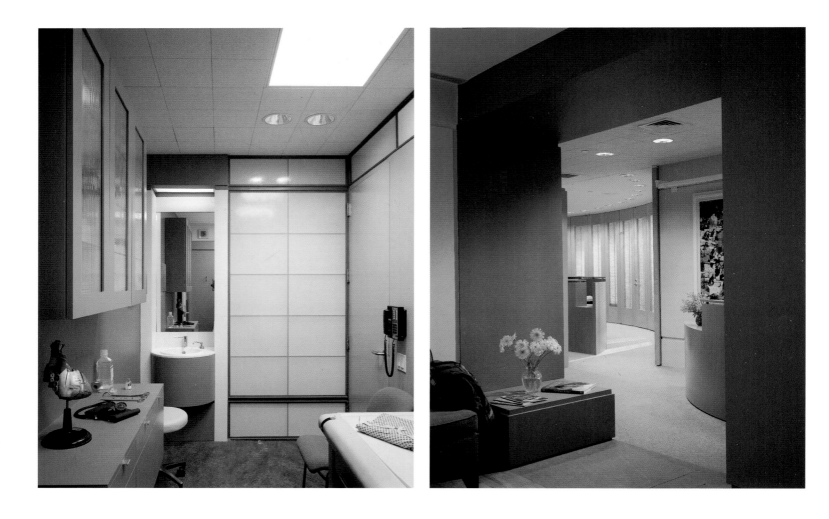

The design team's major concerns were making the Cardiothoracic Surgery division's small space function efficiently and creating a comfortable, calm, noninstitutional environment for patients. The space's semicircular shape made it especially challenging to achieve a graceful fit for the many program elements.

Surgeons' offices along the interior's windowed perimeter are bounded by a continuous arc of glazed doors that pass natural light to the rest of the suite. Two exam rooms support pre- and postsurgery examinations. Administrative and conference spaces are also provided.

The client and design team wanted the suite to have the atmosphere of a private doctor's office instead of a large institution. The color palette, lighting, furniture, finishes, and artwork contribute to an atmosphere that is both warm and professional.

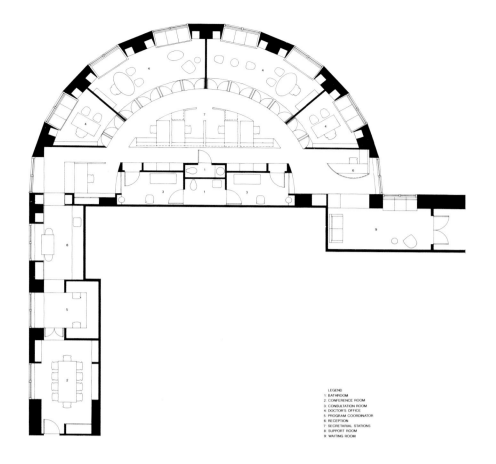

LEGEND
1: BATHROOM
2: CONFERENCE ROOM
3: CONSULTATION ROOM
4: DOCTOR'S OFFICE
5: PROGRAM COORDINATOR
6: RECEPTION
7: SECRETARIAL STATIONS
8: SUPPORT ROOM
9: WAITING ROOM

Owner
Columbia Presbyterian Medical Center

Data

Type of Facility
Ambulatory cardiothoracic care suite

Context
Hospital-based

Type of Construction
Renovation

Area of Project
2,900 GSF

Cost of Construction
$425,000

Cost of Medical Equipment
Not available

Status of Project
Completed July 1993

Credits

Architect
Pasanella + Klein Stolzman + Berg Architects, PC
330 West 42nd Street
New York, New York 10036

Mechanical/Electrical Engineer
H. C. Yu Consulting Engineers
New York, New York

Lighting Consultant
Jerry Kugler Associates, Inc.
New York, New York

Cost Consultants
NASCO Associates, Inc.
New York, New York

Hardware Consultants
Glezen Associates
Elmsford, New York

Art Consulting
Leader Associates
Wayne, New Jersey

Contractor
Herbert Construction Company
New York, New York

Photographer
Chuck Choi
Brooklyn, New York

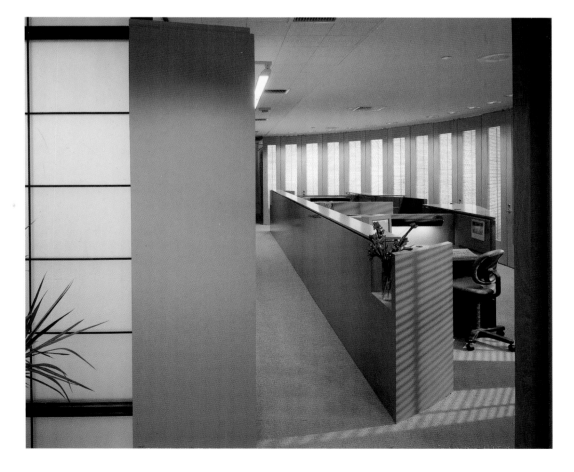

The Denver Health Center

Tulsa, Oklahoma

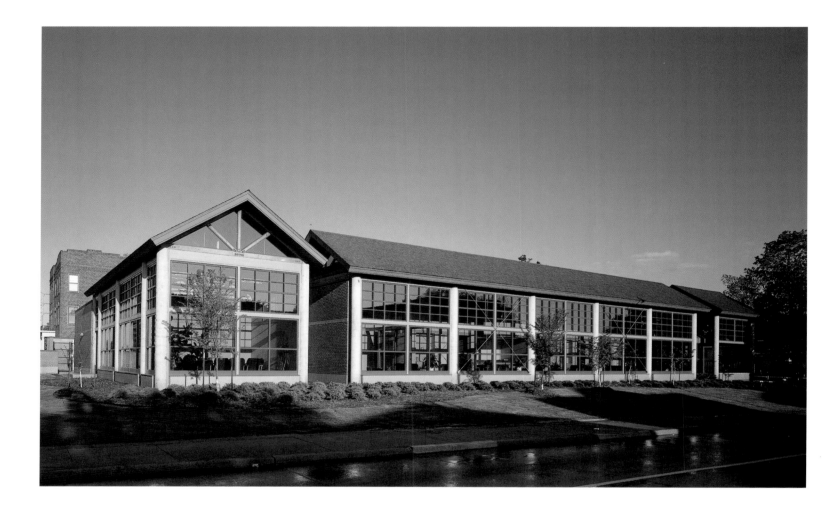

ARCHITECT'S STATEMENT

The design of this six-physician primary care clinic is the result of a straightforward approach to functional relationships and use of space, materials, and daylighting to produce a relaxed environment for patients. The staff areas promote interaction and communication while providing efficient, functional work areas.

The clinic's site at the edge of an older residential neighborhood challenged the design team. The building was divided into two zones: public/staff and clinic/diagnostic. The public/staff areas were broken into residential-scale forms and volumes, while the clinic/diagnostic areas respond to the older multifamily residences that abut the site. The result is a contextual response that supports and strengthens the surrounding neighborhood while providing a therapeutic and interesting environment for patients and staff.

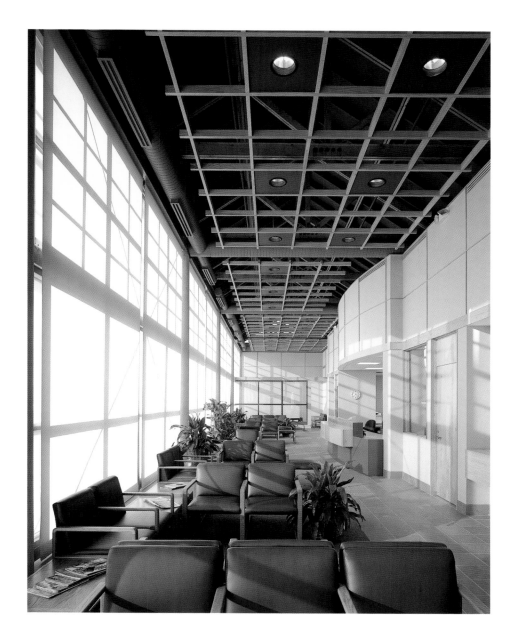

Owner
PruCare/Medical Care Associates of Tulsa

Data

Type of Facility
Primary care clinic

Context
Freestanding

Type of Construction
New

Area of Building
13,308 GSF

Cost of Construction
$1,185,000

Cost of Medical Equipment
$85,000

Status of Project
Completed December 1994

Credits

Architect
Selser Schaefer Architects
1820 South Boulder Avenue,
Suite 300
Tulsa, Oklahoma 74119

Structural Engineer
Wallace Engineering—Structural Consultants
Tulsa, Oklahoma

Mechanical/Electrical Engineer
Flynt & Kallenberger, Inc.
Tulsa, Oklahoma

Landscape Design
Alaback Design Associates
Tulsa, Oklahoma

Contractor
Cowen Construction Company, Inc.
Tulsa, Oklahoma

Photographer
Don Wheeler
Tulsa, Oklahoma

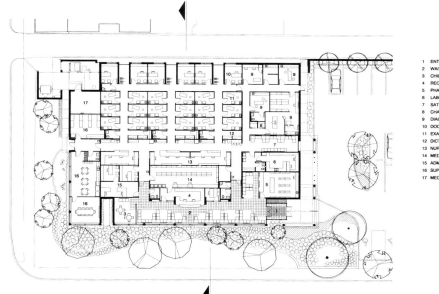

1 ENTRY VESTIBULE
2 WAITING
3 CHILDREN'S WAITING
4 RECEPTION
5 PHARMACY
6 LABORATORY
7 SATELLITE WAITING
8 CHANGING ROOMS
9 DIAGNOSTIC/PROCEDURE ROOMS
10 DOCTOR'S OFFICE
11 EXAM ROOM
12 DICTATION STATION
13 NURSES'S STATION
14 MEDICAL RECORDS
15 ADMINISTATION OFFICES
16 SUPPORT SERVICES
17 MECHANICAL ROOM

FLOOR PLAN

0 2 5   10   20   40

Greater Lawrence Family Health Center, Inc.

Lawrence, Massachusetts

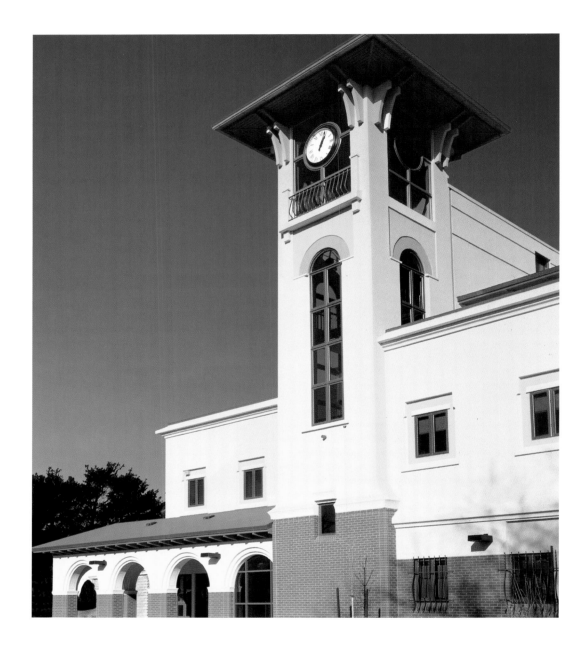

A community health center and family-practice residency program brought health care and doctors to an underserved area. Offered in conjunction with Tufts University and Lawrence General Hospital, the residency program is a national model for training primary care physicians.

Located on the hospital campus, the building was sited to maximize views of the Spicket River and create a courtyard entrance with a pedestrian arcade. A commuter path reinforces the health center's link with the hospital.

In response to the area's Hispanic culture, a mission style was chosen as a precedent for the design. The clock tower recalls the city's important historical buildings. A wayfinding system of arched portals throughout the interior references the architecture in form, color, and materials.

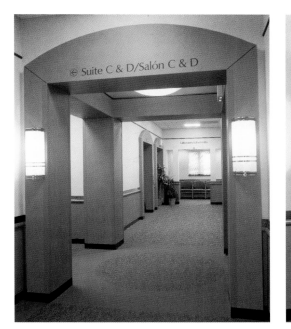

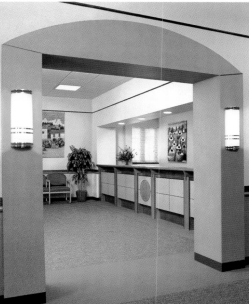

O w n e r

Greater Lawrence Family Health
Center, Inc.

D a t a

Type of Facility

Ambulatory care facility and
family-practice residency program

Context

Freestanding

Type of Construction

New

Area of Building

36,000 GSF

Cost of Construction

$3,500,000

Cost of Medical Equipment

Not available

Status of Project

Completed November 1994

C r e d i t s

Architect

SBA | Steffian Bradley
Associates Inc.
100 North Washington Street
Boston, Massachusetts 02114

Structural Engineer

Charles Chaloff Consulting
Engineer, Inc.
Boston, Massachusetts

Mechanical Engineer

Frank P. DiBiase Associates
Wakefield, Massachusetts

Electrical Engineer

Verne G. Norman Associates, Inc.
South Weymouth, Massachusetts

Geotechnical Engineer

Goldberg-Zoino Associates, Inc.
Newton Upper Falls,
Massachusetts

Civil Engineer

H. W. Moore & Associates, Inc.
Boston, Massachusetts

Contractor

Erland Construction, Inc.
Burlington, Massachusetts

Photographer

John Bellenis
Hamilton, Massachusetts

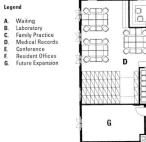

Legend

A. Waiting
B. Laboratory
C. Family Practice
D. Medical Records
E. Conference
F. Resident Offices
G. Future Expansion

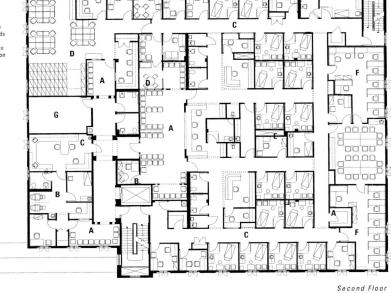

Second Floor

MedPlex

Memphis, Tennessee

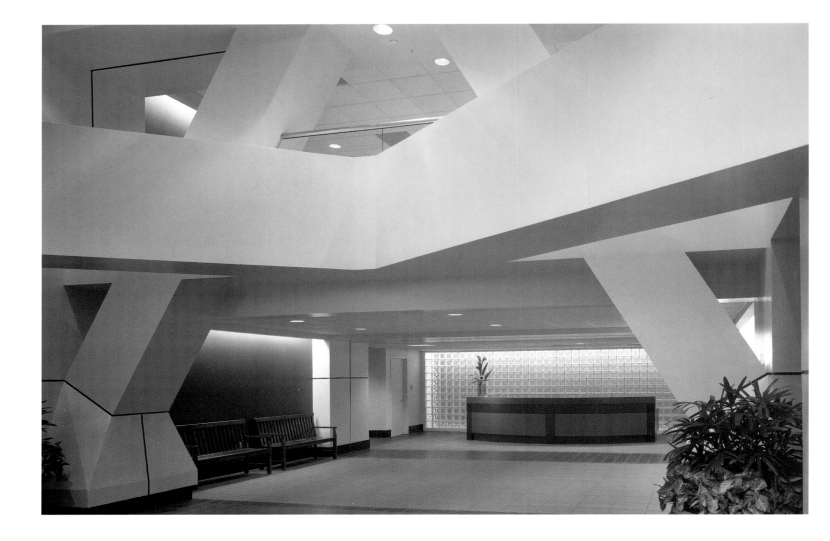

This new ambulatory care center, a replacement for an existing facility, required a high degree of design adaptability to allow building and operational planning to occur simultaneously. Intense collaboration between health care providers and designers was necessary to respond to decisions made during the process that were meant to achieve maximum access to the hospital's complex systems for outpatient diagnostics and treatment.

Unsure of the future direction of health-care reform, the designers used a flexible floor plan that fits well in any kind of delivery system. Clinic floors are designed around shared modules, allowing the facility to absorb the daily patient load without overtaxing staff or patients.

Designers were challenged to find a way to support the teaching of residents at the center while providing an efficient, private model of patient care. The physician teaching spaces are 12-by-24-foot rooms located between each pair of modules. These rooms are used for attending physician/resident conferences and are equipped with computers, telephones, and text materials needed for resident training. Rooms are located so the training functions are not apparent to the patient, eliminating the "specimen under the microscope" feeling many patients experience in traditional resident-training situations.

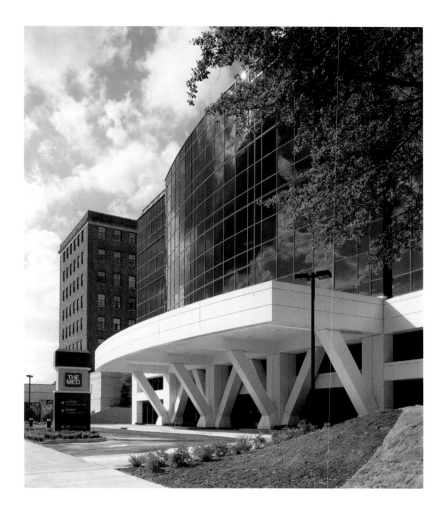

O w n e r
Shelby County Health Care
Corporation

D a t a

Type of Facility
Ambulatory care center

Context
Freestanding

Type of Construction
New

Area of Building
225,973 GSF

Cost of Construction
$18,520,000

Cost of Medical Equipment
$4,325,000

Status of Project
Completed November 1994

C r e d i t s

Architect
JMGR Inc.
80 Monroe Avenue
Memphis, Tennessee 38103

Structural Engineer
Burr and Cole Consulting Engineers
Memphis, Tennessee

Mechanical/Electrical Engineer
JMGR Inc.
Memphis, Tennessee

Consulting Architect
McKissack, McKissack
& Thompson
Memphis, Tennessee

Civil Engineer
Toles & Associates
Memphis, Tennessee

Interior Design
Looney Ricks Kiss Architects
Memphis, Tennessee

Contractor
Turner Construction
Memphis, Tennessee

Photographer
Alan Karchmer
Washington, D.C.

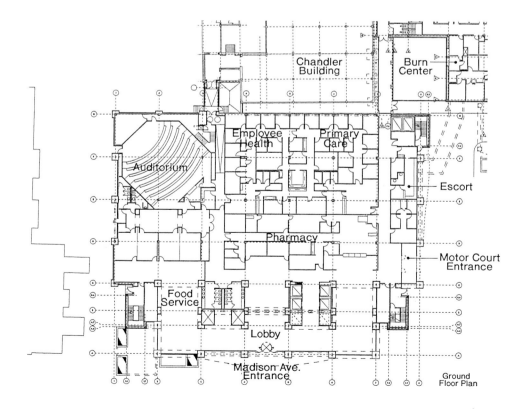

Ground
Floor Plan

MultiCare Medical Center

Tacoma, Washington

Owner

MultiCare Medical Center

Data

Type of Facility

Outpatient center (oncology and imaging), perinatal center, multifloor circulation network, and parking garage

Context

Hospital-based: 450 beds

Type of Construction

New and renovation

Area of Building

215,000 GSF (165,000 new; 50,000 renovation)

Cost of Construction

$35,000,000 ($24,000,000 new construction; $5,000,000 renovation; $6,000,000 garage and plaza)

Cost of Medical Equipment

$2,000,000

Status of Project

Completed September 1994

Credits

Architect

Giffin Bolte Jurgens, p.c.
815 S.W. Second Avenue,
Suite 600
Portland, Oregon 97204

Structural Engineer

Chalker Putnam Collins & Scott
Tacoma, Washington

Mechanical Engineer

Notkin Engineering, Inc.
Seattle, Washington

Electrical Engineer

James D. Graham & Associates, Inc.
Portland, Oregon

Civil Engineers

kpff Consulting Engineers
Seattle, Washington

Vertical Transportation

Lerch Bates Hospital Group, Inc.
Novato, California

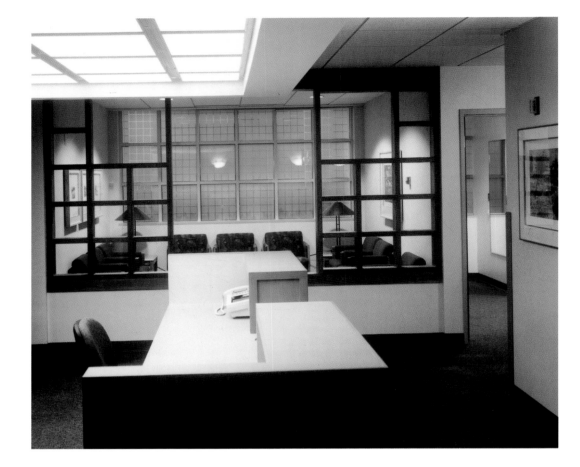

ARCHITECT'S STATEMENT

The project's primary purpose is to provide consolidated facilities for key outpatient services (diagnostic imaging and oncology). Also included are a laboratory, perinatal center, and garage. The outpatient center was built over and around an existing services building and is designed for vertical expansion.

A new vertical/horizontal circulation network links all existing and new hospital areas. An entry plaza was created to bring outpatients directly to the new outpatient center. An interior "street" connects outpatient facilities with all other public areas of the complex. A landscaped fountain courtyard is provided as a separate entrance for radiation therapy patients.

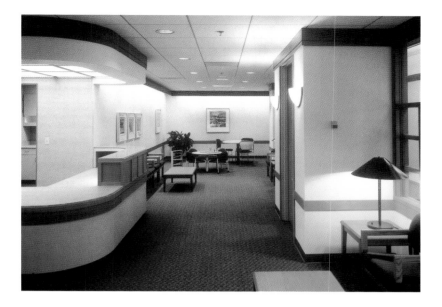

Credits (continued)

Landscape Architecture

Bruce Dees & Associates
Tacoma, Washington

Contractor

Lease Crutcher Lewis
Seattle, Washington

Photographer

Ed Hershberger
Portland, Oregon

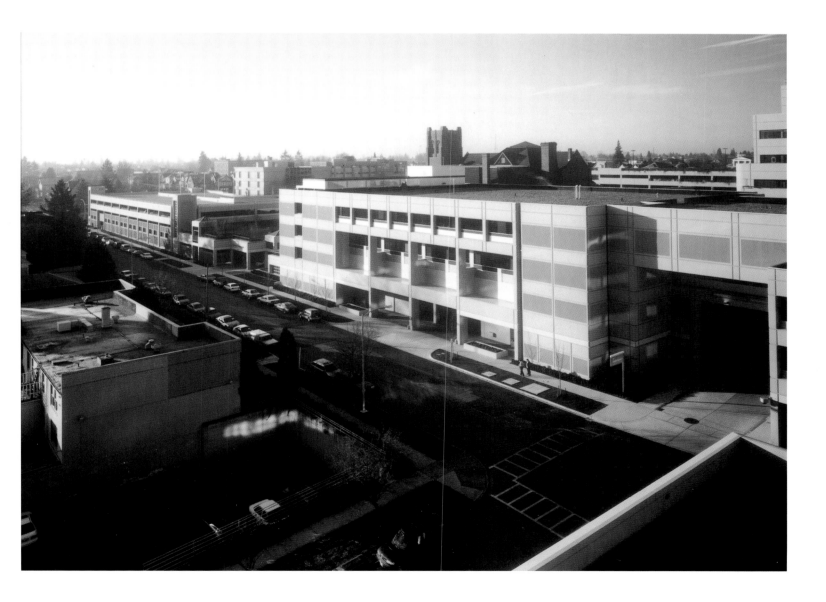

Sutter Avenue Ambulatory Care Facility

Brooklyn, New York

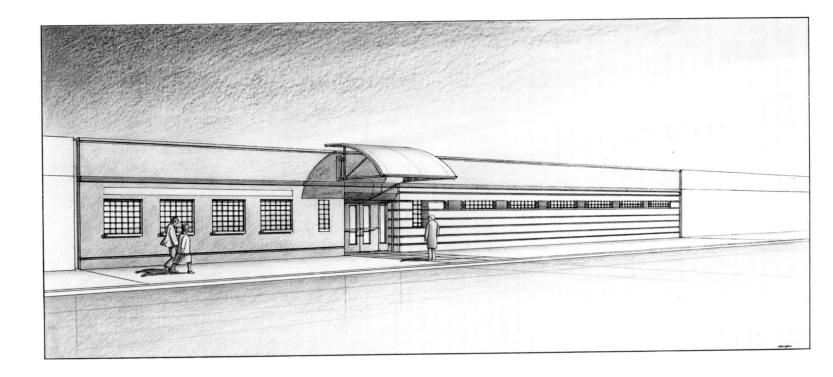

ARCHITECT'S STATEMENT

This ambulatory care center is an outreach clinic for a large metropolitan health care network. Converted from a one-story, 10,000-square-foot former supermarket, it is an example of today's trend toward siting local ambulatory care facilities near activity and population centers.

The design aims to reduce patient stress and create an efficient staff environment. Public and staff entry points are separated and lead into clearly zoned examination and treatment modules. A strongly defined central spine with colorful angled walls on one side facilitates wayfinding, and skylights above key nodes bring healing natural light into the center of the facility.

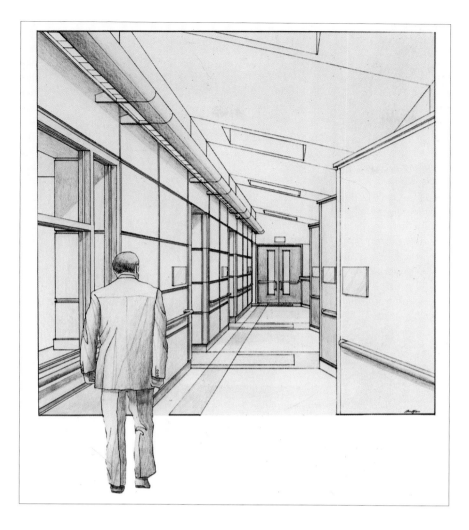

Owner
Catholic Medical Center
of Brooklyn & Queens
Jamaica, New York

Data

Type of Facility
Ambulatory care center

Context
Freestanding

Type of Construction
Renovation

Area of Building
10,000 BGSF

Cost of Construction
Bid estimate: $1,398,150

Medical Equipment Costs
Not available

Status of Project
Estimated completion date:
October 1995

Credits

Architect
Architecture for Health, Science
& Commerce P.C. (AHSC)
777 Old Saw Mill River Road
Tarrytown, New York 10591

Structural Engineer
Severud Associates
New York, New York

Mechanical Engineer
Caretsky & Associates
New York, New York

Contractor
James A. Jennings Co.
Mamaroneck, New York

LEGEND

1. LOBBY / RECEPTION
2. WAITING
3. BUSINESS OFFICE
4. MEDICAL RECORDS
5. SOCIAL WORKER
6. NUTRITIONIST & HEALTH EDUCATION
7. SUB-WAITING
8. PHLEBOTOMY / SPECIMEN
9. EXAM ROOM
10. CONSULTATION
11. SONOGRAM
12. RADIOLOGY
13. MAMMOGRAM
14. CONFERENCE ROOM
15. ADMINISTRATIVE OFFICE
16. STAFF LOUNGE / LOCKERS
17. SOILED HOLDING
18. CLEAN HOLDING

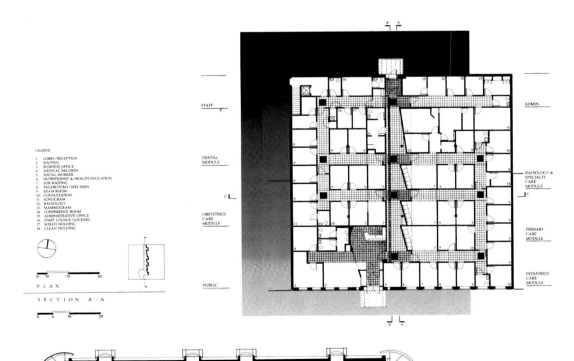

PLAN

SECTION A - A

The Takopid Health Center

Tacoma, Washington

Owner
>   The Puyallup Tribal Health Authority

Data
>   *Type of Facility*
>   Ambulatory care medical center
>   and dental clinic
>
>   *Context*
>   Freestanding
>
>   *Type of Construction*
>   New
>
>   *Area of Building*
>   36,576 GSF
>
>   *Construction Costs*
> $4,800,000
>
>   *Medical Equipment Costs*
> $2,100,000
>
>   *Status of Project*
>   Completed September 1993

Credits
>   *Architect*
>   The Tsang Partnership, Inc.
>   1221 Second Avenue, Suite 330
>   Seattle, WA 98101
>
>   *Structural Engineer*
>   Chalker, Putnam, Collins &
>   Scott, Inc.
>   Tacoma, Washington
>
>   *Mechanical Engineer*
>   de Montigny Engineers, Inc.
>   Kent, Washington
>
>   *Electrical Engineer*
>   Bouillon Christofferson & Schairer
>   (BCS)
>   Seattle, Washington
>
>   *Civil Engineer*
>   Daley Engineering Co.
>   Kent, Washington
>
>   *Landscape Architect*
>   Gail Staeger Associates
>   Seattle,Washington
>
>   *Interior Designer*
>   Bonnie Aaby, Designs Unlimited
>   Bellingham, Washington
>
>   *Cost Estimator*
>   Matson Carlson & Associates, Inc.
>   Seattle, Washington

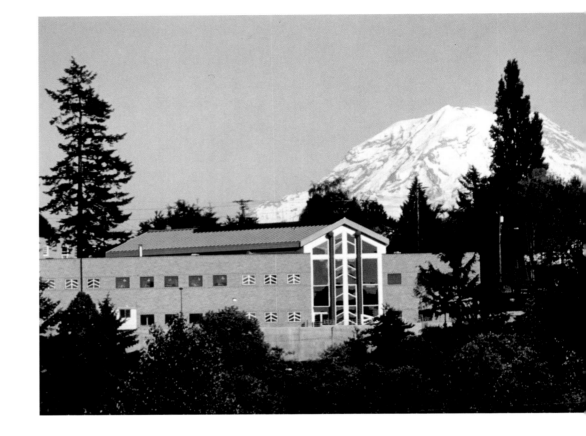

ARCHITECT'S STATEMENT

With Mt. Rainier as its backdrop, the Takopid Health Center sits majestically on a steeply graded site overlooking Puyallup Tribal Headquarters. Designed to be expressive of the people it serves, the new ambulatory care center provides health services to an estimated 20,000 Native Americans. The Native American theme resonates throughout the complex in the traditional basket-weave patterns in the brick facade, the sculptured brick salmon designs decorating the front entrance walls, and the longhouse skeletal structure and house post found inside. Integrating art with architecture, the facility celebrates the heritage of the Pacific Northwest Indian.

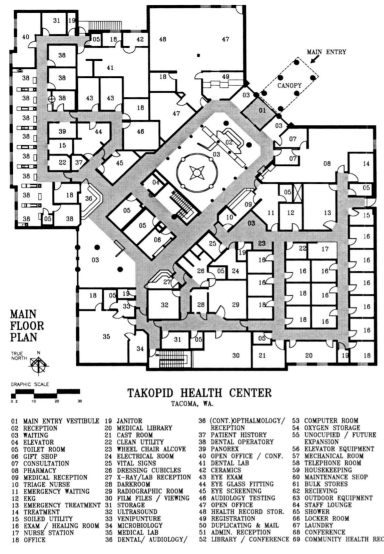

MAIN FLOOR PLAN

TRUE NORTH

N

GRAPHIC SCALE

0 2   10   20   30

TAKOPID HEALTH CENTER
TACOMA, WA.

01 MAIN ENTRY VESTIBULE	19 JANITOR	36 (CONT.)OPTHALMOLOGY/	53 COMPUTER ROOM
02 RECEPTION	20 MEDICAL LIBRARY	RECEPTION	54 OXYGEN STORAGE
03 WAITING	21 CAST ROOM	37 PATIENT HISTORY	55 UNOCCUPIED / FUTURE
04 ELEVATOR	22 CLEAN UTILITY	38 DENTAL OPERATORY	EXPANSION
05 TOILET ROOM	23 WHEEL CHAIR ALCOVE	39 PANOREX	56 ELEVATOR EQUIPMENT
06 GIFT SHOP	24 ELECTRICAL ROOM	40 OPEN OFFICE / CONF.	57 MECHANICAL ROOM
07 CONSULTATION	25 VITAL SIGNS	41 DENTAL LAB	58 TELEPHONE ROOM
08 PHARMACY	26 DRESSING CUBICLES	42 CERAMICS	59 HOUSEKEEPING
09 MEDICAL RECEPTION	27 X-RAY/LAB RECEPTION	43 EYE EXAM	60 MAINTENANCE SHOP
10 TRIAGE NURSE	28 DARKROOM	44 EYE GLASS FITTING	61 BULK STORES
11 EMERGENCY WAITING	29 RADIOGRAPHIC ROOM	45 EYE SCREENING	62 RECIEVING
12 EKG	30 FILM FILES / VIEWING	46 AUDIOLOGY TESTING	63 OUTDOOR EQUIPMENT
13 EMERGENCY TREATMENT	31 STORAGE	47 OPEN OFFICE	64 STAFF LOUNGE
14 TREATMENT	32 ULTRASOUND	48 HEALTH RECORD STOR.	65 SHOWER
15 SOILED UTILITY	33 VENIPUNTURE	49 REGISTRATION	66 LOCKER ROOM
16 EXAM / HEALING ROOM	34 MICROBIOLOGY	50 DUPLICATING & MAIL	67 LAUNDRY
17 NURSE STATION	35 MEDICAL LAB	51 ADMIN. RECEPTION	68 CONFERENCE
18 OFFICE	36 DENTAL/ AUDIOLOGY/	52 LIBRARY / CONFERENCE	69 COMMUNITY HEALTH RECEPTION

Credits (continued)

Carver/Artist

Jay Haavik
Seattle, Washington

Contractor

Donald M. Drake Company
Portland, Oregon

Photographers

Robert G. Weisenbach, AIA
Seattle, Washington

Jeff Schroeder
Tacoma, Washington

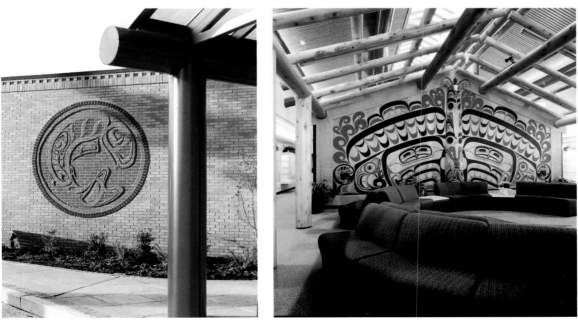

Department of Veterans Affairs/VA Outpatient Clinic

Los Angeles, California

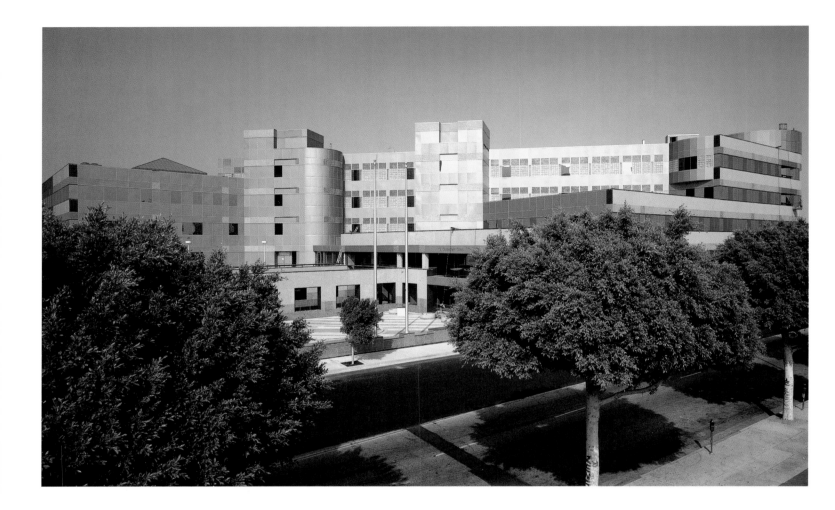

ARCHITECT'S STATEMENT

Located at the eastern edge of Los Angeles's busy civic center, the clinic provides two million veterans with medical, surgical, psychiatric, and rehabilitation spaces. The design is sensitive to the needs of the clientele at this outpatient clinic with anticipated daily attendance of more than 700. The clinic architecture is a visually stimulating synthesis of opposing forces: urban density and open space; federal and industrial design; granite and metal surfaces; horizontal and vertical axes; and high-technology clinics and humane spaces.

The western fenestration is articulated with a pattern of translucent glass blocks, reflective of traditional shoji screens found in the adjacent community of Little Tokyo. The windows allow protected light to enter the main circulation spines.

From the paved automobile court and entry of the outpatient clinic, a series of gardens step through the building. Parking terrace, roof gardens, and an interior atrium encourage pedestrian activity, which is further reinforced by a streetside arcade that connects with the building entry. Entrance and frontal orientation align with the dominant downtown building grid that organizes the civic center. The patterns continue through the clinic's organization with the location of public, administrative, and general offices.

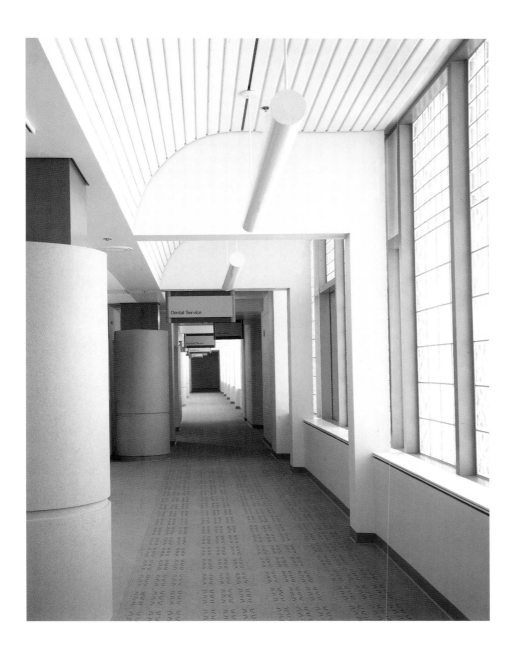

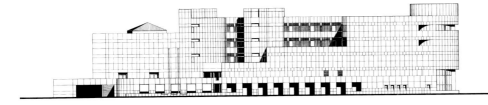

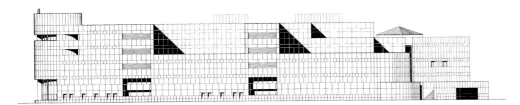

Owner
Department of Veterans Affairs

Data
Type of Facility
Health care/public project/ outpatient clinic

Context
Freestanding

Type of Construction
New

Area of Building
340,000 GSF

Cost of Construction
$48,000,000

Cost of Medical Equipment
Not available

Status of Project
Completed August 1992

Credits
Architect
Bobrow/Thomas and Associates (BTA)
1001 Westwood Boulevard
Los Angeles, California 90024

Structural Engineer
CYGNA Consulting Engineer
Marina Del Rey, California

Mechanical/Electrical Engineer
Hayakawa Associates, Consulting Engineers
Los Angeles, California

Specifications Consultant
PROSPEC
Tehachapi, California

Acoustical Design
Paul S. Veneklasen and Associates
Santa Monica, California

Exterior Wall Design
Horvath & Associates, Inc.
Chicago, Illinois

Contractor
J. W. Bateson
Los Angeles, California

Photographer
Michael Arden
Sherman Oaks, California

University of Washington Medical Center
Roosevelt Ambulatory Care Center

Seattle, Washington

O w n e r
University of Washington
Alumni Association

D a t a

Type of Facility
Outpatient care facility

Context
Freestanding

Type of Construction
New

Area of Building
94,877 GSF

Cost of Construction
$16,813,000

Cost of Medical Equipment
$7,390,000

Status of Project
Completed October 1994

C r e d i t s

Architect
NBBJ
111 South Jackson Street
Seattle, Washington 98104

Structural Engineer
kpff Consulting Engineers
Seattle, Washington

Mechanical Engineers
Chamberlain Mechanical
Corporation
Kirkland, Washington

MacDonald-Miller Company, Inc.
Seattle, Washington

Electrical Engineers
McKinney & Associates
Kirkland, Washington

Veca Electric
Bellevue, Washington

Cochran
Seattle, Washington

Equipment Planner
NBBJ
Seattle, Washington

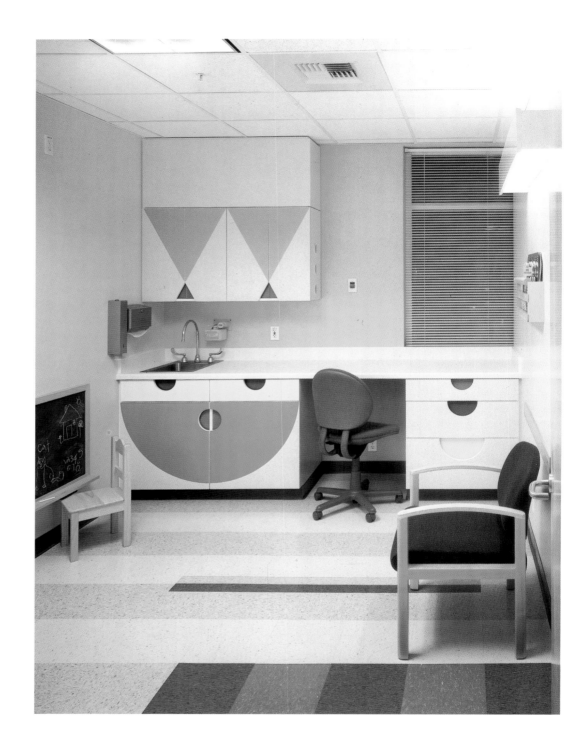

1. Lobby
2. Reception
3. Pharmacy
4. Lab
5. Admin.

6. Invetro Fertilization Lab
7. Medical Records
8. Offices
9. Loading Dock
10. Material Management

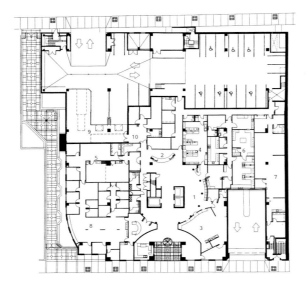

Credits (continued)

Cost Consultant
NBBJ
Seattle, Washington

Contractor
GLY Construction
Seattle, Washington

Photographer
Doug Walker
Olympia, Washington

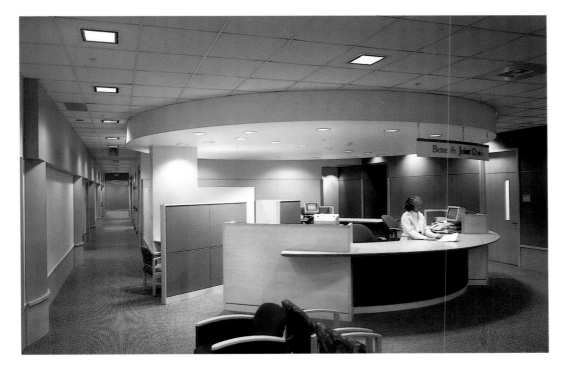

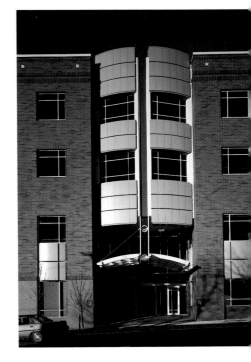

ARCHITECT'S STATEMENT

Designed for the University of Washington Medical Center, this four-story outpatient care facility houses a laboratory, medical records, a pharmacy, and centers for bone and joint care, exercise training, family medicine, fertility and endocrine services, imaging, internal medicine, a pain clinic, pediatrics, and women's care. The building balances highly advanced systems such as teleradiology and fiber optics with an environment softened and humanized by design, color, and materials. Fitting comfortably into its residential neighborhood, the brick-clad building represents an interpretation of Collegiate Gothic, borrowing architectural details from 1920s apartment houses nearby, as well as from the older University of Washington campus.

West Allis Memorial Hospital Ambulatory Care Facility

West Allis, Wisconsin

Owner
West Allis Memorial

Data

Type of Facility
Ambulatory care

Context
Hospital-based: 70 beds

Type of Construction
New and renovation

Area of Building
174,800 GSF
(138,000 new; 36,800 renovation)

Cost of Construction
$29,756,922
($21,709,981 new; $8,046,941
renovation)

Cost of Medical Equipment
$2,600,000

Status of Project
Completed June 1994

Credits

Architect
Flad & Associates
644 Science Drive, P.O. Box 44977
Madison, Wisconsin 53744-4977

Structural Engineer
Flad Structural Engineers
Madison, Wisconsin

Mechanical/Electrical Engineer
Affiliated Engineers, Inc.
Madison, Wisconsin

Geotechnical Engineer
Woodward-Clyde
Milwaukee, Wisconsin

Acoustics Consultant
Yerges Acoustics
Woodbridge, Illinois

Planning Consultant
Space Diagnostics
Madison, Wisconsin

Contractors
General Construction:
CG Schmidt, Inc.
Milwaukee, Wisconsin

Electrical Construction:
Staff Electric Co., Inc.
Menomonee Falls, Wisconsin

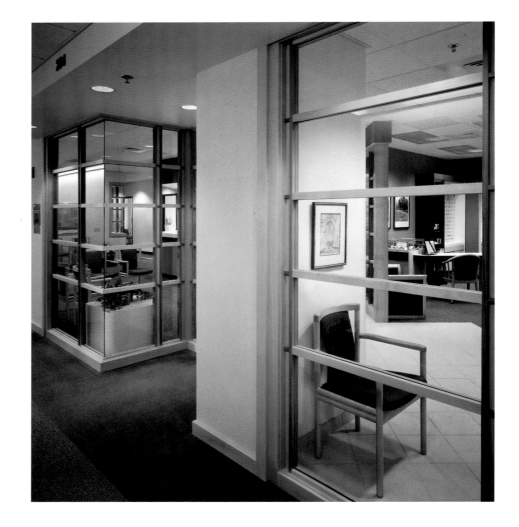

ARCHITECT'S STATEMENT

The facility enhances hospital operations while offering a healing, pleasing environment for patients, hospital staff, and the surrounding community. With the strategic vision of providing cost-effective health care to this suburban community, the architect addressed several issues: providing physicians' offices, expanding the ambulatory care facility and surgery suite, allowing for additional parking, and creating a cohesive image for the entire facility. These goals were met by creating a hospital campus centered around a courtyard that serves as a focal point and unifying element.

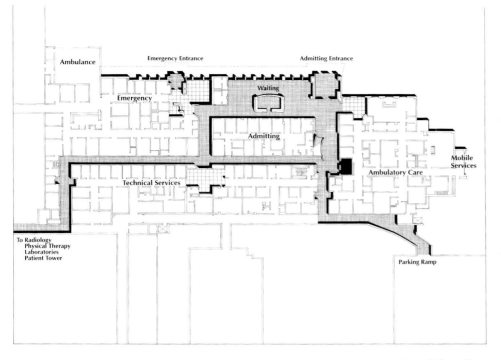

Ambulance

Emergency Entrance

Admitting Entrance

Emergency

Waiting

Admitting

Mobile
Services

Technical Services

Ambulatory Care

To Radiology
Physical Therapy
Laboratories
Patient Tower

Parking Ramp

Ground Floor Plan

Credits (continued)
Mechanical/Plumbing Construction:
Wenninger Company, Inc.
New Berlin, Wisconsin

Photographers
Harr, Hedrich-Blessing
Chicago, Illinois

Joe Paskus
Madison, Wisconsin

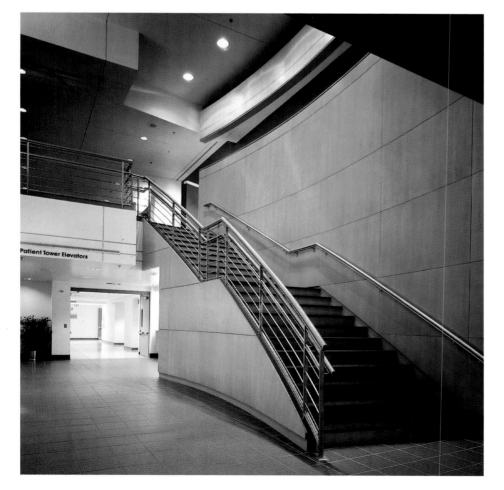

Patient Tower Elevators

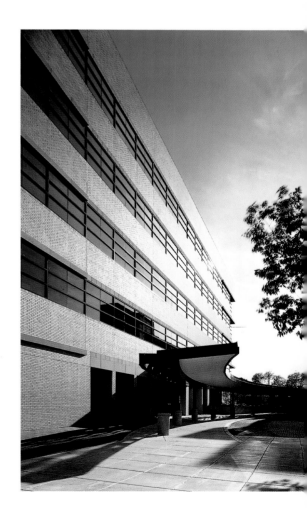

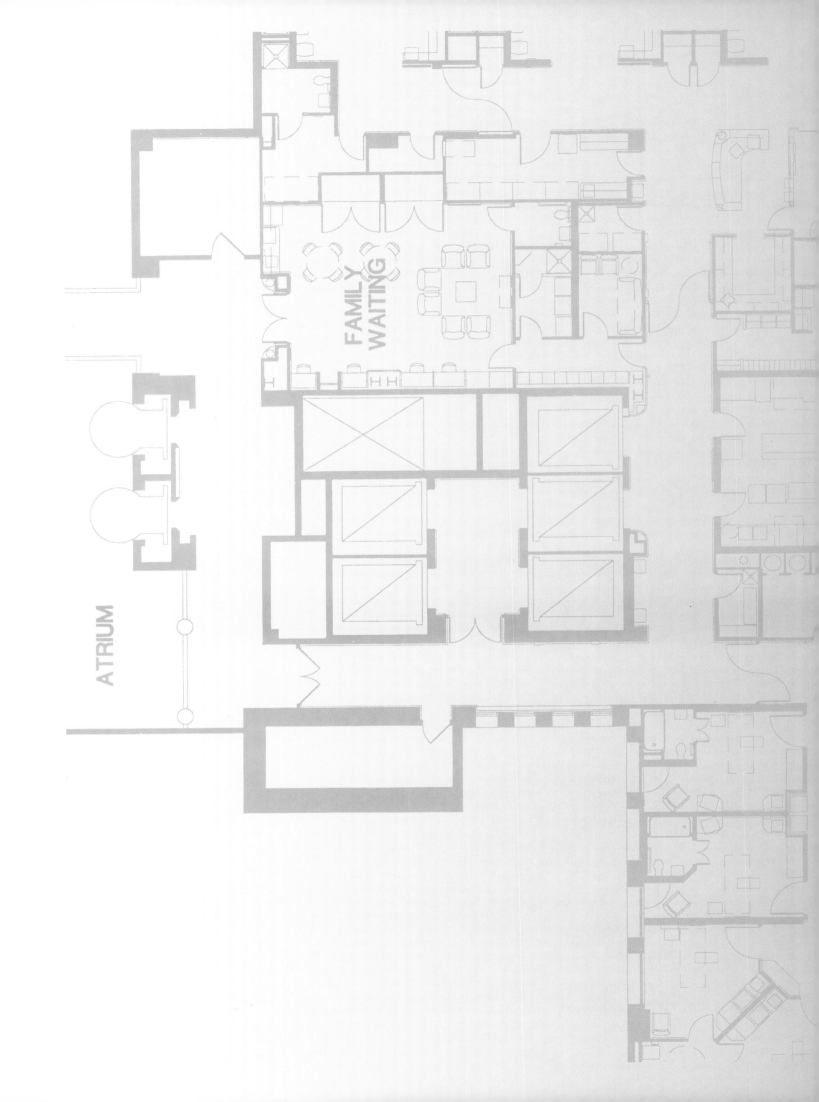

Cancer Centers

BONE MARROW TRANSPLANT UNIT

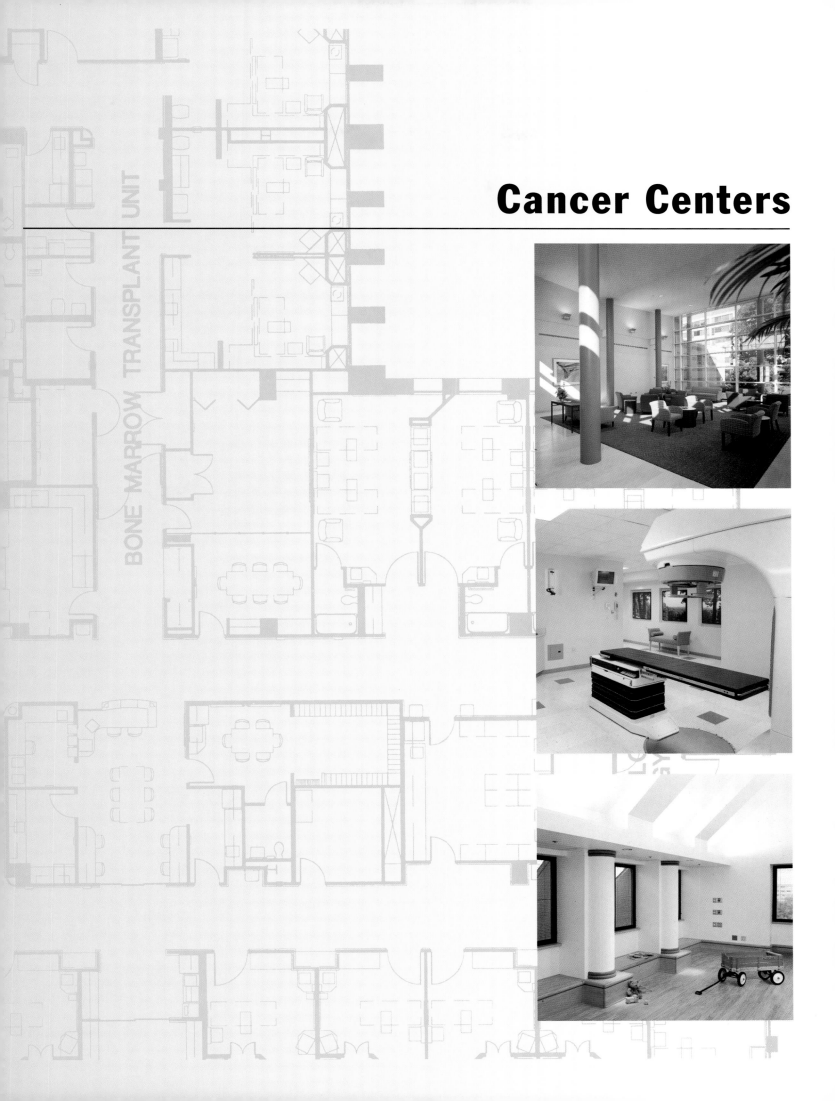

Bloomington Regional Cancer Center

Bloomington, Indiana

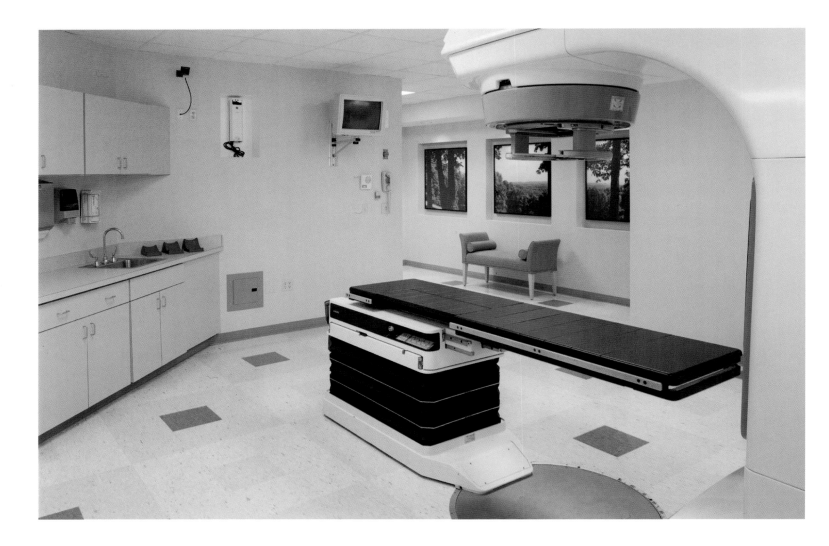

ARCHITECT'S STATEMENT

The challenge of designing a high-tech facility within a low budget was met through construction methods and research of building materials and equipment. A concrete/wood framed structure, brick, and exterior insulation finish system created the cost-efficient design. In addition, the floor plan design allowed for efficient use of space by cancer patients and staff members. The linear accelerator rooms are located in the high-tech zone toward the back of the facility and are integrated into the natural landscape of the site.

Natural light, elegant finishes, and views to the outside were the main elements used to establish a comforting and welcoming environment for patients.

These elements are featured throughout the facility and reinforced by the incorporation of the central courtyard. The courtyard connects all but a few spaces to the outdoors, allowing patients to experience the benefits of natural light.

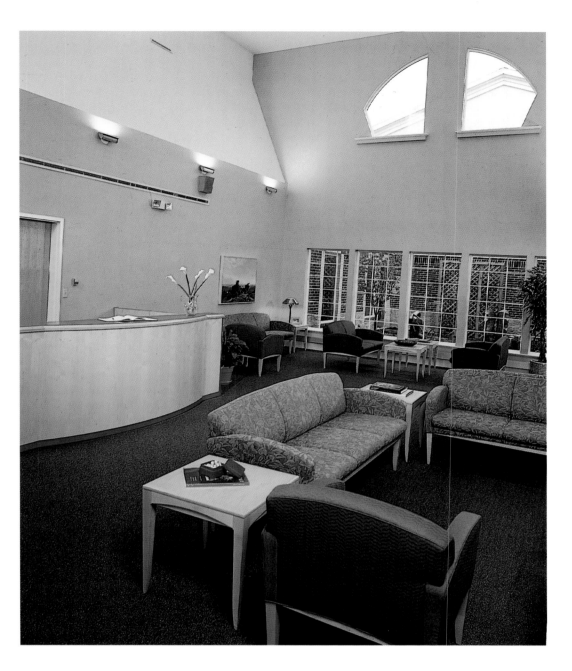

Owner
Bloomington Hospital

Data

Type of Facility
Cancer center

Context
Freestanding

Type of Construction
New

Area of Building
12,000 GSF

Cost of Construction
$1,500,000

Cost of Medical Equipment
Not available

Status of Project
Completed July 1994

Credits

Architect
BSA Design
6810 North Shadeland Avenue
Indianapolis, Indiana 46220

Structural / Mechanical / Electrical Engineer
BSA Design
Indianapolis, Indiana

Contractor
Hokanson Companies, Inc.
Indianapolis, Indiana

Photographer
Mardan Photography
Indianapolis, Indiana

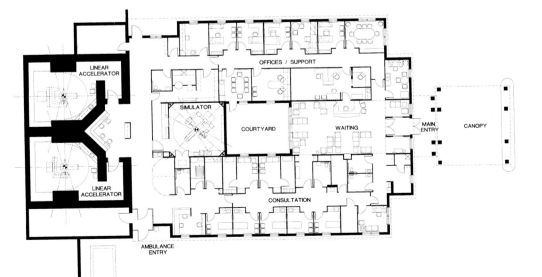

The Children's Cancer Center—James Whitcomb Riley Hospital for Children

Indianapolis, Indiana

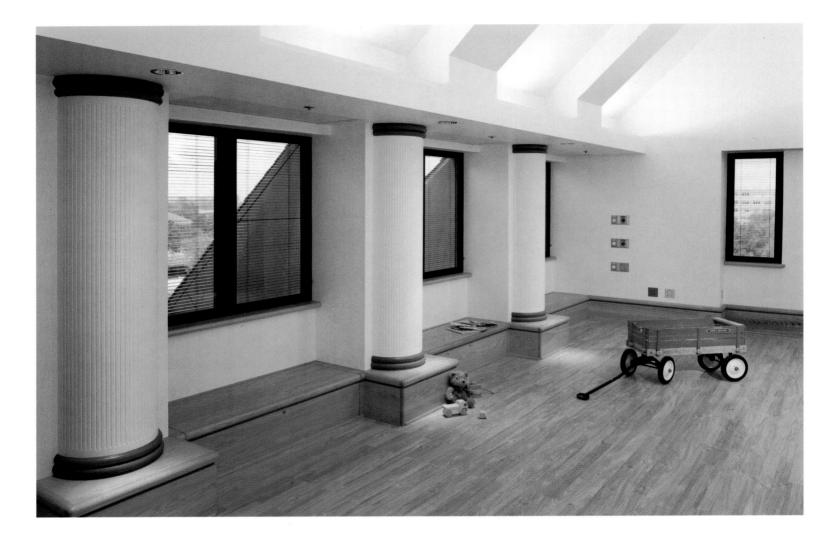

ARCHITECT'S STATEMENT

The new Children's Cancer Center, a fifth-floor addition to the James Whitcomb Riley Hospital for Children, serves as the pediatric inpatient component for the Indiana University Cancer Program, providing services for hematology/oncology patients and bone marrow transplant patients. The center was also designed to work in conjunction with the Herman B. Wells Center for Pediatric Research.

The challenge of establishing a color palette acceptable to various age levels was achieved by using a modified primary color scheme and a more sophisticated secondary color palette. The use of wood throughout the space added warmth for the patients' benefit in addition to functionality and durability for the client's benefit. Natural lighting above the main nurse's station and indirect lighting above patient room doors add variation and interest throughout the center.

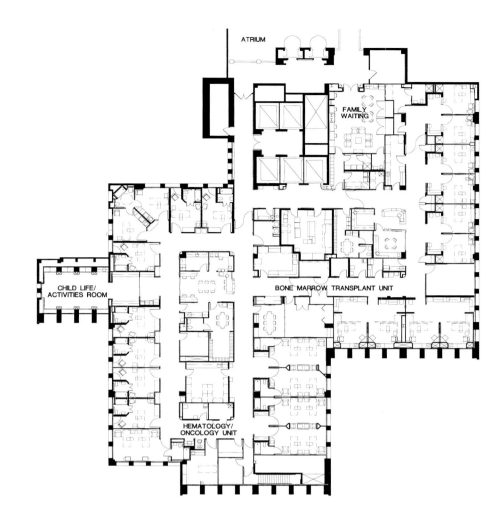

ATRIUM

FAMILY WAITING

CHILD LIFE/ ACTIVITIES ROOM

BONE MARROW TRANSPLANT UNIT

HEMATOLOGY/ ONCOLOGY UNIT

Owner
Indiana University Hospitals

Data

Type of Facility
Pediatric cancer center

Context
Hospital-based: 30 beds

Type of Construction
New

Area of Building
23,700 GSF

Cost of Construction
$6,032,900

Cost of Medical Equipment
Not available

Status of Project
Completed November 1993

Credits

Architect
BSA Design
6810 North Shadeland Avenue
Indianapolis, Indiana 46220

Structural/Mechanical/Electrical Engineer
BSA Design
Indianapolis, Indiana

Contractor
Huber, Hunt & Nichols, Inc.
Indianapolis, Indiana

Photographer
Mardan Photography
Indianapolis, Indiana

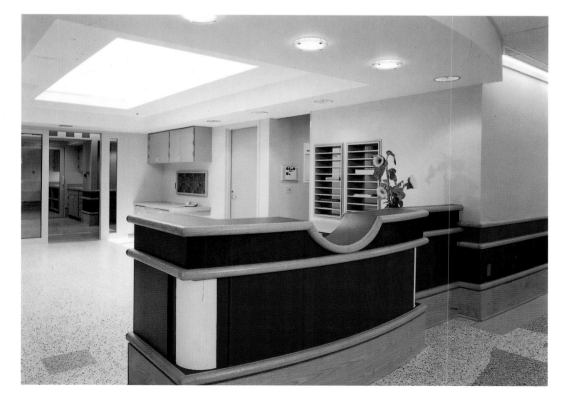

Lakeshore Area Radiation Oncology Center

Holland, Michigan

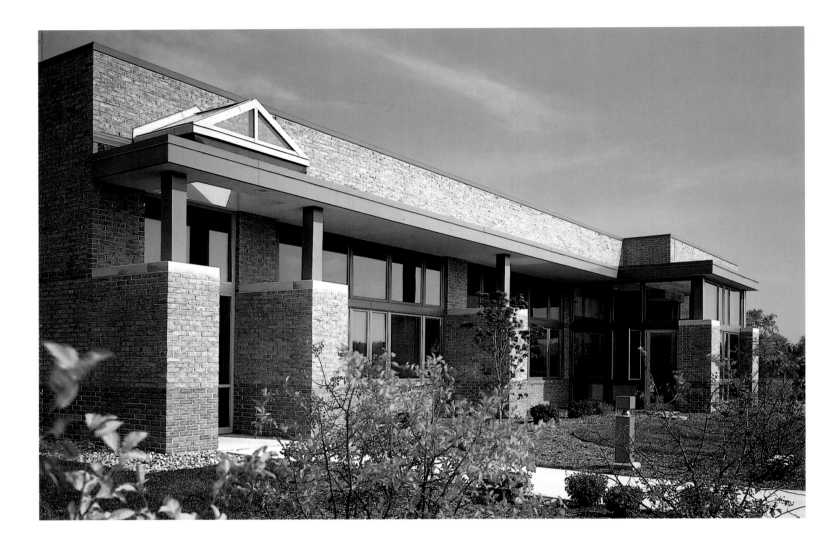

ARCHITECT'S STATEMENT

Four independent hospitals formed a consortium to develop this radiation/oncology treatment facility to serve a fast-growing patient group. The mission was to design a functional but noninstitutional site and facility. The patients' comfort was of primary importance; the architecture was designed to provide a healing and comforting environment. Materials and colors were selected to reflect the soothing atmosphere of Michigan's west coast shoreline. Sand-mold brick, tinted glass, bleached wood trim, and floor/wall coverings in blue-greens, whites, and tans imitate the sand, sky, and water of nearby Lake Michigan. Landscaping materials reinforce an informal setting with freeform grass areas, wildflower edges, and beach grasses.

The facility incorporates a Siemens MEVATRON KDS2 linear accelerator, with plans to add a second accelerator at a later date. A Siemens MEVASIM S simulator is centrally located between the examination, treatment, and physicist work areas. The current and future needs for exam rooms, professional staff offices, and support spaces are incorporated.

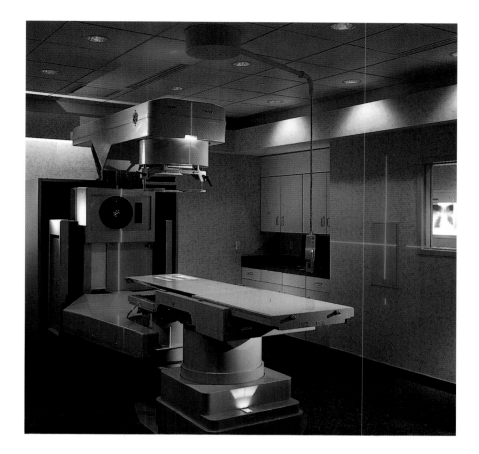

Owner
Lakeshore Radiation Oncology
Consortium

Data
Type of Facility
Consortium-owned radiation/
oncology treatment center

Context
Freestanding

Type of Construction
New

Area of Building
10,300 GSF

Cost of Construction
$1,400,000

Cost of Medical Equipment
$1,775,000

Status of Project
Completed June 1993

Credits
Architect
Greiner, Inc.
3950 Sparks Drive, SE
Grand Rapids, Michigan 49546

*Structural/Mechanical/Electrical
Engineer*
Greiner, Inc.
Grand Rapids, Michigan

Contractor
Muskegon Construction Company
Muskegon, Michigan

Photographer
Gary Quesada
Korab/Hedrich Blessing
Troy, Michigan

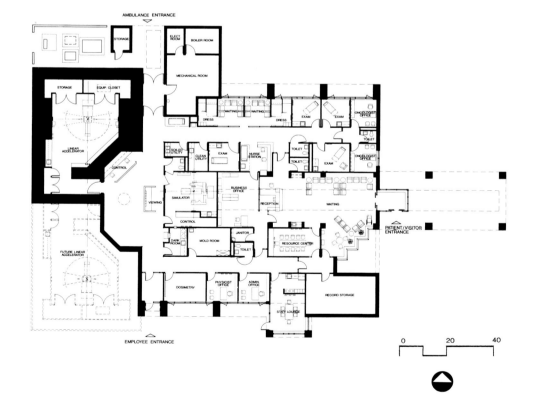

John and Dorothy Morgan Cancer Center

Allentown, Pennsylvania

Owner
Lehigh Valley Hospital

Data

Type of Facility
Comprehensive ambulatory cancer
management center

Context
Hospital-based: No beds

Type of Construction
New

Area of Building
156,200 GSF

Cost of Construction
$19,800,000

Cost of Medical Equipment
$4,500,000

Status of Project
Completed November 1993

Credits

Architect
TRO/The Ritchie Organization
80 Bridge Street
Newton, Massachusetts 02158

Structural Engineer
Foley and Buhl Engineers, Inc.
Watertown, Massachusetts

*Mechanical/Electrical/Plumbing/Fire
Protection Engineer*
Gillian & Hartmann, Inc.
Valley Forge, Pennsylvania

Civil Engineer
G. Edwin Pidcock Co.
Allentown, Pennsylvania

Medical Suite Architect
Howard Kulp Architects
Allentown, Pennsylvania

Planner
TRO/The Ritchie Organization
Newton, Massachusetts

Interior Designer
TRO/The Ritchie Organization
Newton, Massachusetts

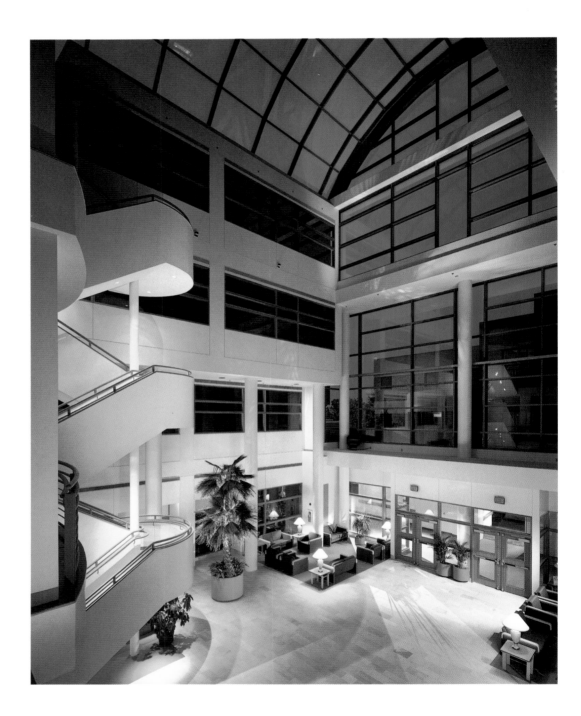

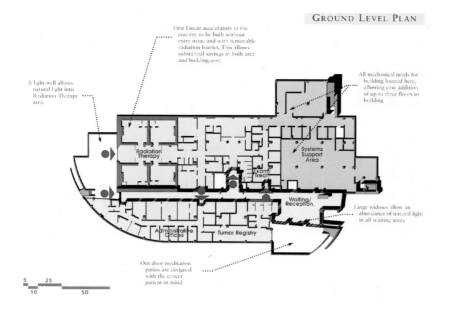

First Linear accelerators in the country to be built without entry maze and with removable radiation barrier. This allows substantial savings in built area and building cost.

A light-well allows natural light into Radiation Therapy area.

All mechanical needs for building located here, allowing easy addition of up to three floors to building

Radiation Therapy

Systems Support Area

Exam/Treat

Waiting/Reception.

Large widows allow an abundance of natural light in all waiting areas

Administrative Offices

Tumor Registry

Out door meditation patios are designed with the cancer patient in mind

5   25
10   50

Credits (continued)
Landscape Architect
  McCloskey & Faber, P.C.
  Horsham, Pennsylvania

Construction Manager
  Alvin H. Butz, Inc.
  Allentown, Pennsylvania

Photographers
  Warren Jagger
  Providence, Rhode Island

  Don Pearse
  Springfield, Pennsylvania

  Steven Wolfe
  Bethlehem, Pennsylvania

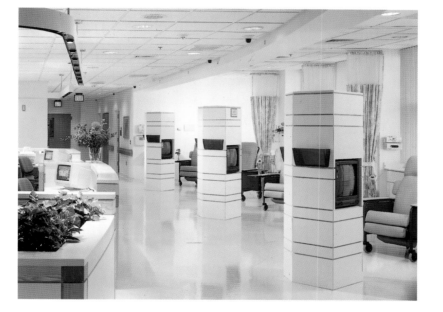

ARCHITECT'S STATEMENT

The new Lehigh Valley Cancer Center and Ambulatory Care Pavilion intertwines technology with healing. The four-story building was designed to expand vertically to eight stories. In addition to this flexibility to grow, the interior planning of the building was designed for change. For instance, the radiation shielding at linear accelerator vaults is removable, so that radiation therapy can eventually be replaced by a future treatment methodology without the leftover physical constraints typical of concrete linac vaults.

Aside from the very sophisticated technology employed in the project, the building's most unique aspect is that it is actually two buildings with distinct entrances: one for cancer care and the other for routine diagnostics and physician access. This allows operational efficiencies without compromising patient convenience.

The Marjorie G. Weinberg Cancer Care Center

Melrose Park, Illinois

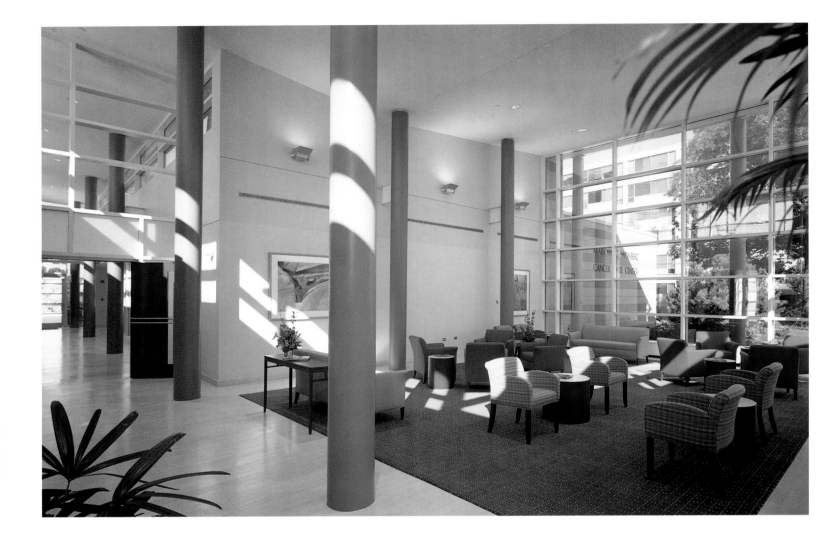

The hospital's strategic plan called for creation of a facility that would provide a feeling of hope and a sense of inspiration. The client wanted to reduce the fragmentation of oncology care by combining medical and radiation oncology into one facility. It was extremely important that the center meet the community needs for oncology as they relate to prevention, treatment, education, and emotional support. Finally, they wanted to develop a facility capable of providing state-of-the-art treatment today and in future years.

The synthesis of architecture, furnishings, and landscape design creates a peaceful setting for this new, patient friendly cancer care center. A freestanding building on a hospital campus, the center is among the most technologically advanced of its kind and is designed to accommodate both medical and radiation therapy. This facility includes a 21 MEV linear accelerator, simulation equipment and support areas for radiation treatment, an eight-room clinic, and a medical oncology treatment area.

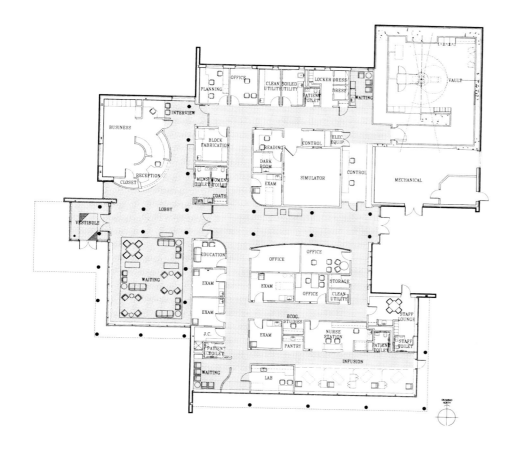

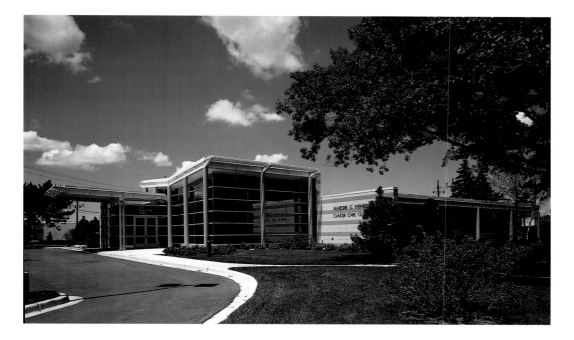

Owner

Gottlieb Community Health
Services

Data

Type of Facility

Cancer care center

Context

Freestanding

Type of Construction

New

Area of Building

14,400 GSF

Cost of Construction

$2,000,000

Cost of Medical Equipment

Not available

Status of Project

Completed November 1993

Credits

Architect

Loebl Schlossman and Hackl, Inc.

Interior Architect

LSH/Hague-Richards Associates
Chicago, Illinois

Structural Engineer

Rittweger & Tokay, Inc.
Park Ridge, Illinois

Mechanical/Electrical Engineer

Robert G. Burkhardt & Associates
Chicago, Illinois

Civil Engineer

SDI Consultants, Ltd.
Oak Brook, Illinois

Landscape Architect

Paul Vett
Wheaton, Illinois

Contractor

The George Sollitt Construction
Company
Wood Dale, Illinois

Photographer

James Steinkamp
Steinkamp/Ballogg Photography
Chicago, Illinois

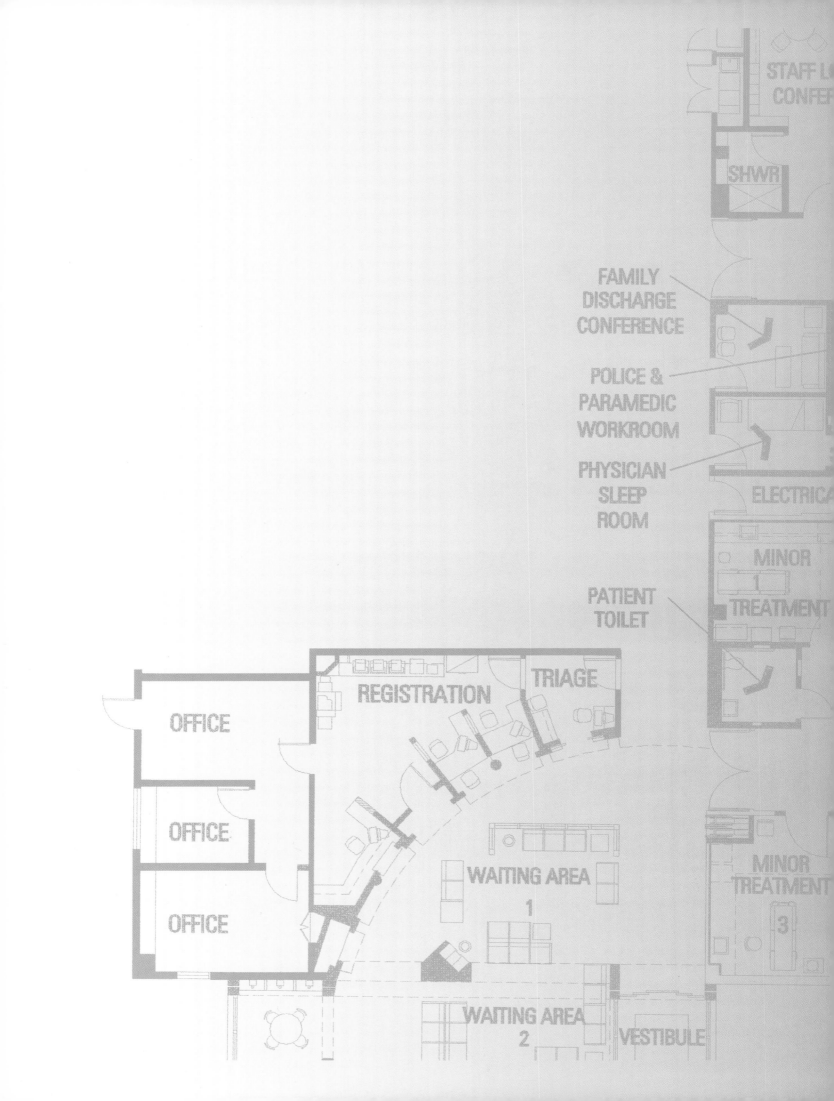

STAFF L
CONFE

SHWR

FAMILY
DISCHARGE
CONFERENCE

POLICE &
PARAMEDIC
WORKROOM

PHYSICIAN
SLEEP
ROOM

ELECTRICA

MINOR
1
TREATMENT

PATIENT
TOILET

TRIAGE

REGISTRATION

OFFICE

OFFICE

OFFICE

WAITING AREA

1

MINOR
TREATMENT

3

WAITING AREA

2

VESTIBULE

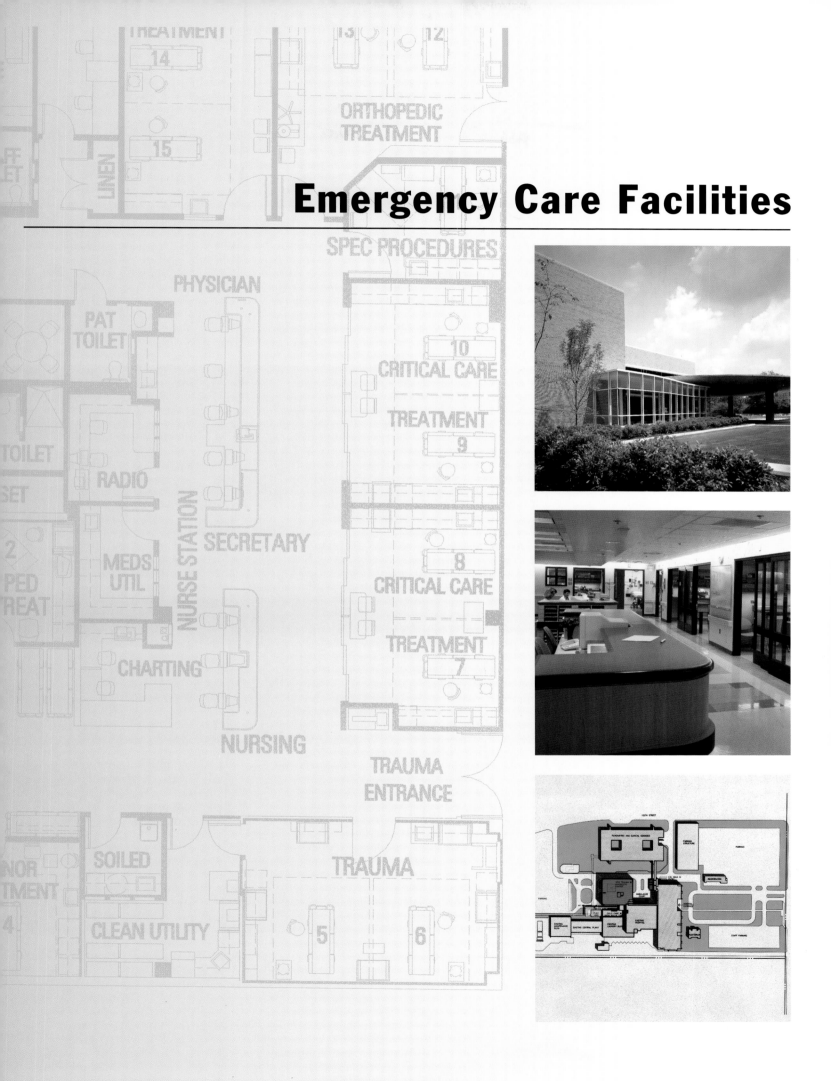

TREATMENT
14

15

LINEN

13   12

ORTHOPEDIC
TREATMENT

Emergency Care Facilities

SPEC PROCEDURES

PHYSICIAN

PAT
TOILET

TOILET

RADIO

MEDS
UTIL

CHARTING

NURSE STATION

SECRETARY

NURSING

10
CRITICAL CARE

TREATMENT
9

8
CRITICAL CARE

TREATMENT
7

TRAUMA
ENTRANCE

2
PED
TREAT

NOR
TMENT

4

SOILED

CLEAN UTILITY

TRAUMA

5   6

Emergency Services Department/Trauma Center
John Muir Medical Center

Walnut Creek, California

Citation

This smaller-scaled project was intriguing in its careful approach to phasing, and in working with a clearly defined set of existing conditions and constraints. A critical department such as emergency and trauma is difficult to maintain in full operation during renovation without such precautions. Some of the existing constraints of the department were improved with minor adjustment (waiting space, imaging capacity, nurse's station), while the capacity of the facility was increased 50 percent with only a small increase in area.

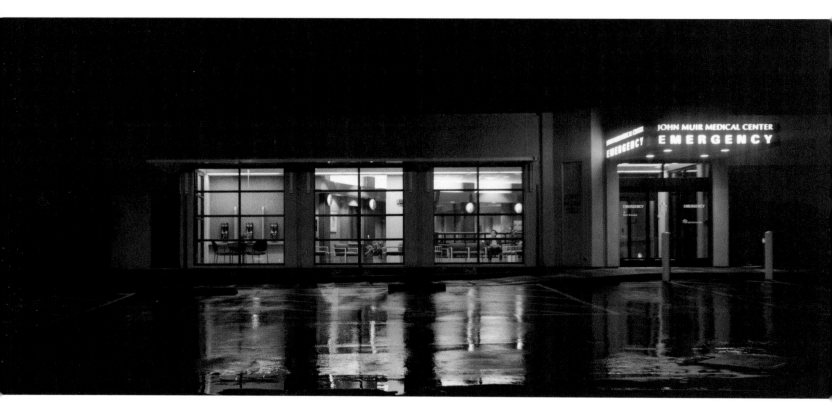

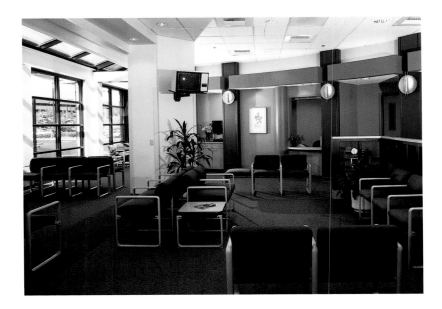

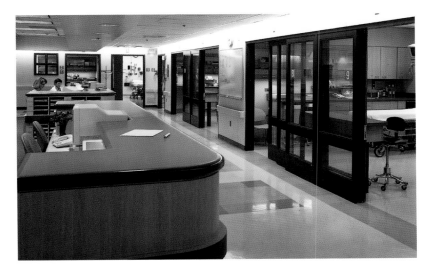

Owner
John Muir Medical Center

Data
Type of Facility
Emergency services

Context
Hospital-based: 343 beds

Type of Construction
Renovation

Area of Building
8,368 GSF (477 new; 7,891
renovation)

Cost of Construction
$1,085,240 ($62,000 new;
$1,023,240 renovation)

Cost of Medical Equipment
$340,000

Status of Project
Completed April 1994

Credits
Architect
Thistlethwaite Architectural Group
250 Sutter Street, Suite 500
San Francisco, California 94108

Structural Engineer
The Sear Brown Group
San Francisco, California

Mechanical Engineer
Ted Jacob Engineering Group, Inc.
Oakland, California

Electrical Engineer
Cammissa and Wipf Consulting
Engineers
San Francisco, California

Civil Engineer
George S. Nolte & Associates
Walnut Creek, California

Medical Physicist
Darlene Belmonte, M.S.
Walnut Creek, California

Contractor
Pozzo Construction Company
Pleasant Hill, California

Photographer
Stephen Fridge
San Francisco, California

ARCHITECT'S STATEMENT

As the regional trauma center serving 885,000 residents, the 343-bed John Muir Medical Center needed to increase the number of treatment stations in the emergency department by 50 percent, accommodate new imaging technology in the existing two-bed trauma room, and increase seating capacity in the waiting area.

The Medical Center treats approximately 1,200 trauma patients and 27,000 emergency patients annually. In order to keep the busy departments fully functional during the in-place remodeling and expansion, the project involved extensive coordination of four phases of construction. It was a program requirement to maintain a minimum of ten treatment stations (two of which were trauma stations) during each phase of construction.

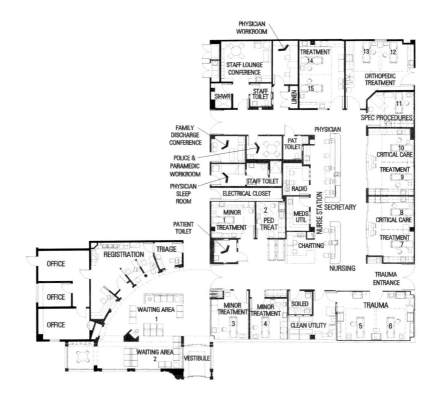

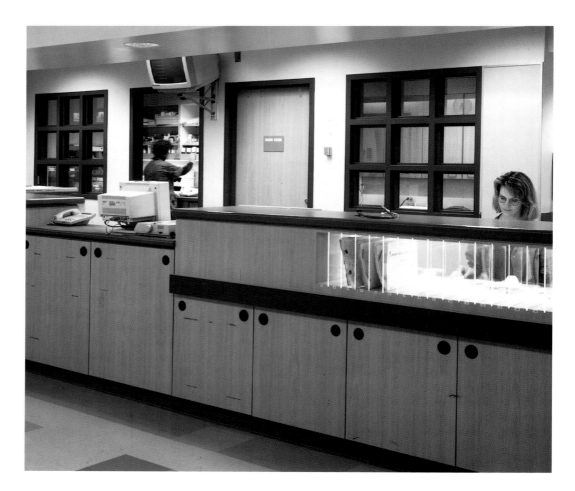

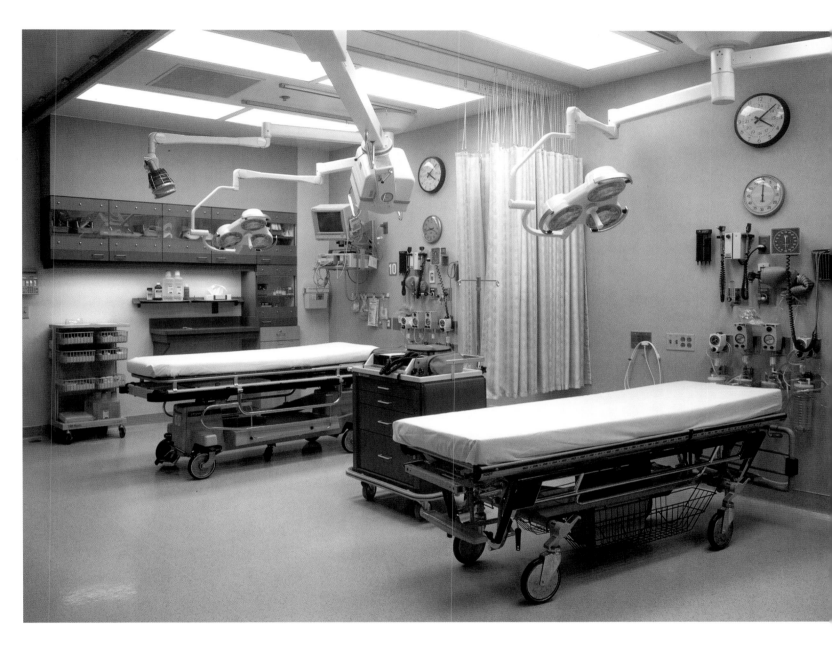

Martin Luther King, Jr./Charles R. Drew Medical Center Trauma Care & Diagnostic Imaging Center

Los Angeles, California

Owner

County of Los Angeles, Department of Health Services

Data

Type of Facility

Trauma care and diagnostic imaging center

Context

Hospital-based: 24 beds

Type of Construction

New

Area of Building

180,000 GSF

Cost of Construction

$42,939,000

Cost of Medical Equipment

$15,600,000

Status of Project

Estimated completion date: March 1996

Credits

Architects

Joint Venture:

Langdon Wilson Architecture Planning Interiors
1055 Wilshire Boulevard, Suite 1500
Los Angeles, California 90017

Kennard Design Group Architecture and Planning
3600 Wilshire Boulevard, Suite 1820
Los Angeles, California 90010

Structural Engineer

John A. Martin & Associates
Los Angeles, California

Mechanical Engineer

Rosenberg & Associates
Los Angeles, California

Electrical Engineer

Patsaouras & Associates
Sherman Oaks, California

Seismic Isolation Consultant

Base Isolation Consultants, Inc.
San Francisco, California

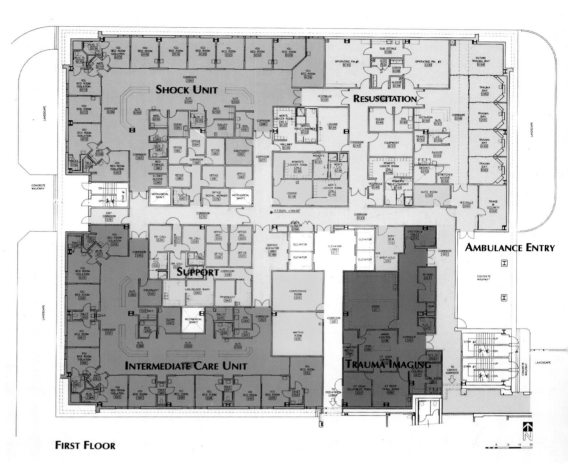

FIRST FLOOR

ARCHITECT'S STATEMENT

The Trauma Care Center will function in addition to the existing Emergency Department. All patients with traumatic injuries will be brought to the Resuscitation Unit of the Trauma Center, where initial critical treatment will be provided. The intent is that all care required by the trauma patient be provided within this facility, including any surgery necessary to save the patient's life. Once the patient has been treated, he or she will be transferred into one of the two-bed units for recovery. The Shock Unit will handle the most acute patients, while the Intermediate Care Unit will handle patients who are relatively stable but still recovering. Patients will be discharged directly from the Trauma Center.

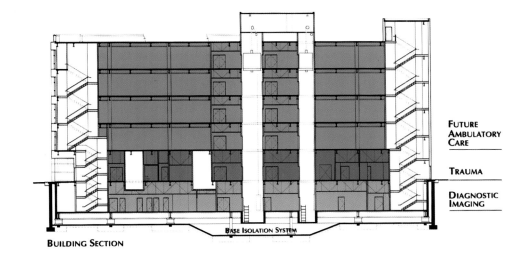

FUTURE
AMBULATORY
CARE

TRAUMA

DIAGNOSTIC
IMAGING

BASE ISOLATION SYSTEM

BUILDING SECTION

C r e d i t s (c o n t i n u e d)

Medical Equipment Planning Consultant

> Facilities Development Inc.
> Phoenix, Arizona

Contractor

> Centex Golden Construction Company
> San Diego, California

Photographer

> Building:
> Warren Aerial Photography, Inc.
> Pacoima, California

> Base Isolators:
> Langdon Wilson Architecture Planning Interiors
> Los Angeles, California

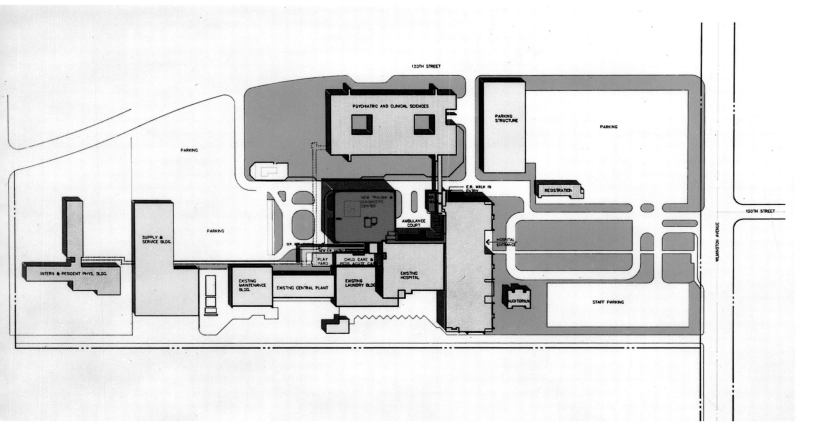

St. Mary's Health Center Emergency Department

St. Louis, Missouri

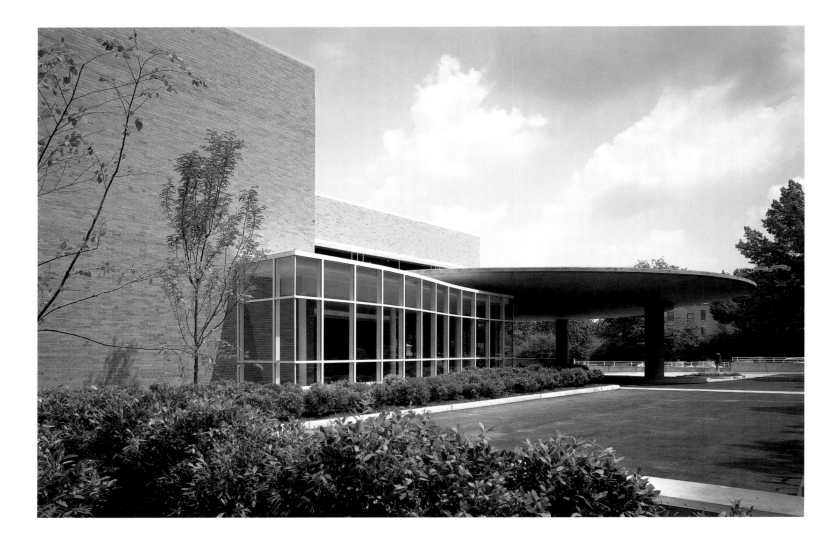

ARCHITECT'S STATEMENT

The new emergency department sets the tone for Project 2000, a five-year, $41 million master facility plan to expand and modernize St. Mary's Health Center. The facility provides 18 treatment rooms. There are special facilities for OB/GYN patients, a decontamination room to treat chemical exposures, multiple registration areas for faster service, "fast track" areas for non-urgent patient care, and a family consultation room.

The layout provides easy access and visual control to all treatment rooms from one central nurses' station. Ten-foot wide corridors provide space for smooth circulation. According to the state architect for the Missouri Department of Health, "What I look for in most projects is clarity of circulation. I've asked my staff to tour St. Mary's emergency room as an example of how good circulation is supposed to be accomplished."

The final product, which came in under budget, was a truly collaborative effort. According to St. Mary's patient-care manager, "By the time the ER was built, everyone on the staff knew exactly what it would look like and what to expect. . . . I wouldn't change a thing."

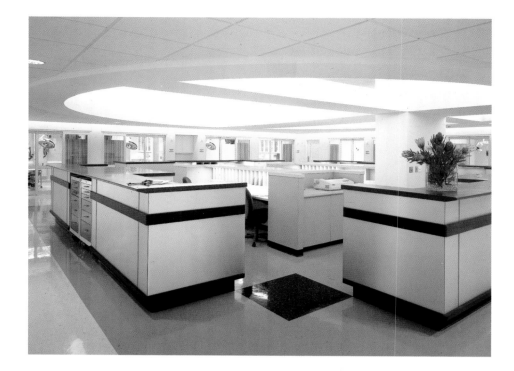

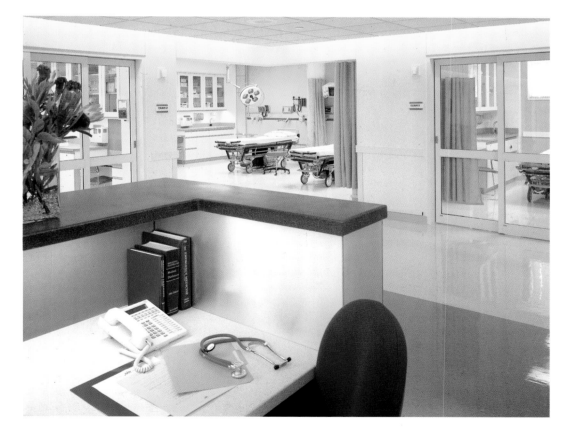

O w n e r
St. Mary's Health Center

D a t a

Type of Facility
Emergency department

Context
Hospital-based: 18 emergency/
3 holding beds

Type of Construction
New

Area of Building
14,000 GSF

Cost of Construction
$4,157,533

Cost of Medical Equipment
$56,445

Status of Project
Completed June 1994

C r e d i t s

Architect
Mackey Mitchell Associates
800 St. Louis Union Station
St. Louis, Missouri 63103

Structural Engineer
Siebold, Sydow & Elfanbaum
St. Louis, Missouri

Mechanical/Electrical Engineer
McGrath, Inc.
St. Louis, Missouri

Health Care Programming Consultant
Tchoukaleff Kelly Associates
St. Louis, Missouri

Lighting Consultant
LAM Partners, Inc.
Cambridge, Massachusetts

Construction Manager
J. S. Alberici Construction Company
St. Louis, Missouri

General Contractor
C. Rallo Contracting Co., Inc.
St. Louis, Missouri

Photographer
Alise O'Brien
St. Louis, Missouri

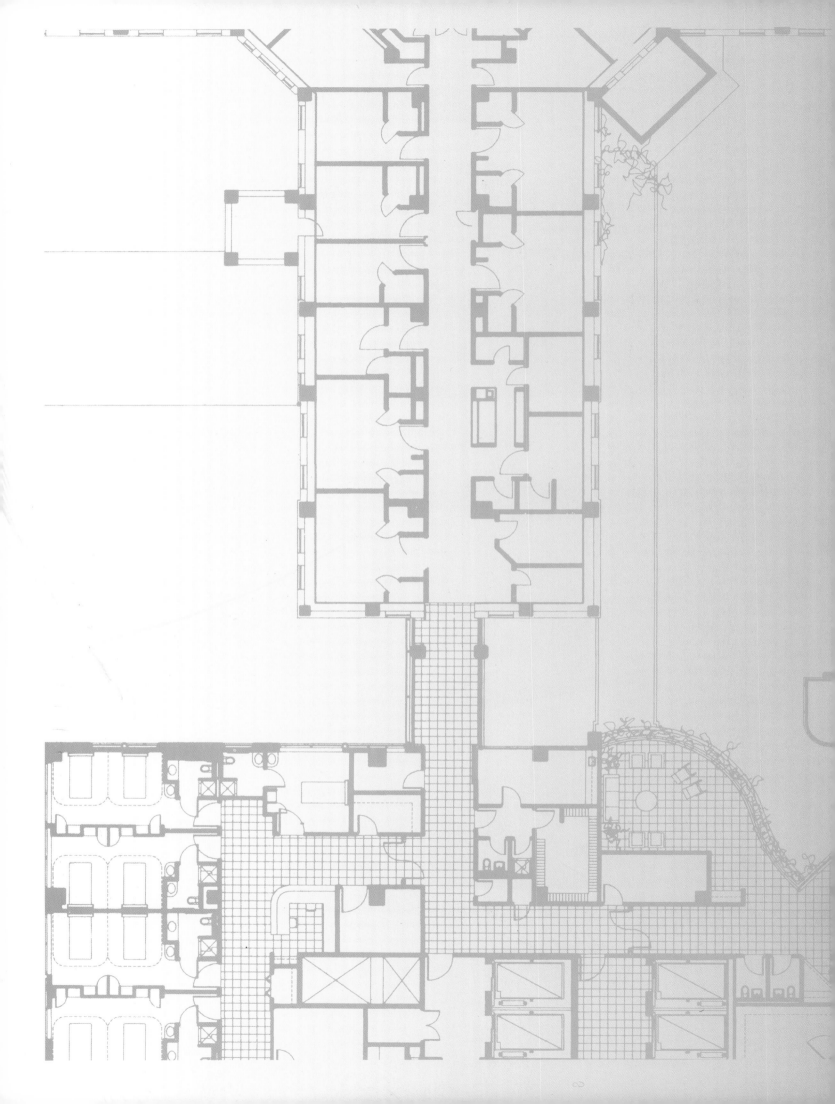

Hospitals and Medical Centers

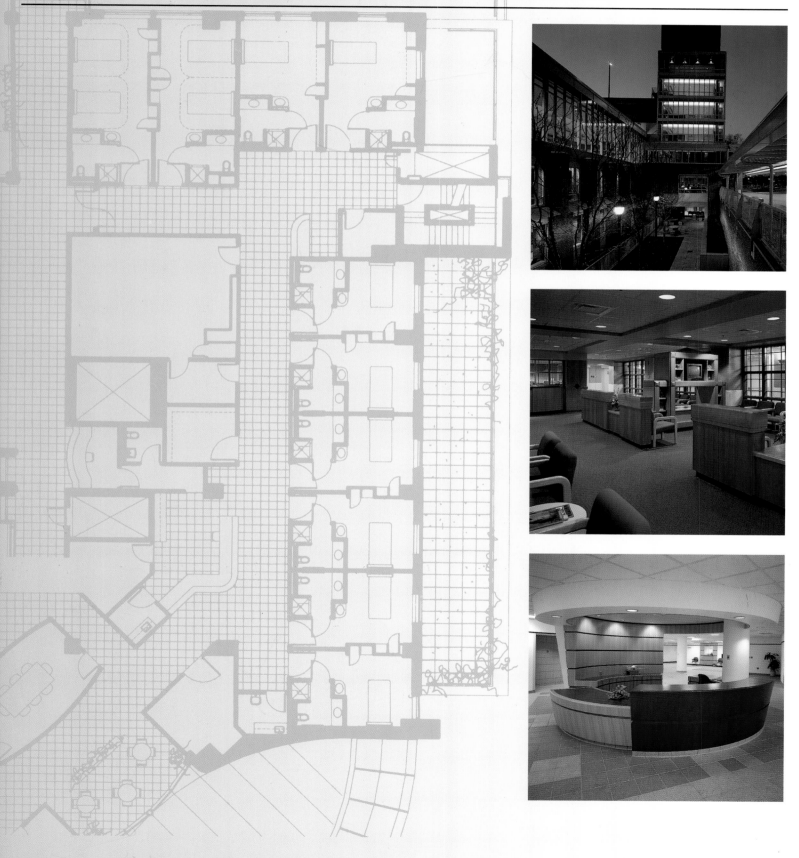

Health Central

Ocoee, Florida

Citation

The brightly colored "pieces and parts" that distinguish the exterior of this playful and exuberant medical center belie the logical and rational development of the overall plan. The integration of a mid-sized hospital with retail and physician office space is seamless and flexible. The program indicated a conscious effort to challenge the user's notion and expectations of a health care facility—and this facility does exactly that, with an exciting and intriguing design.

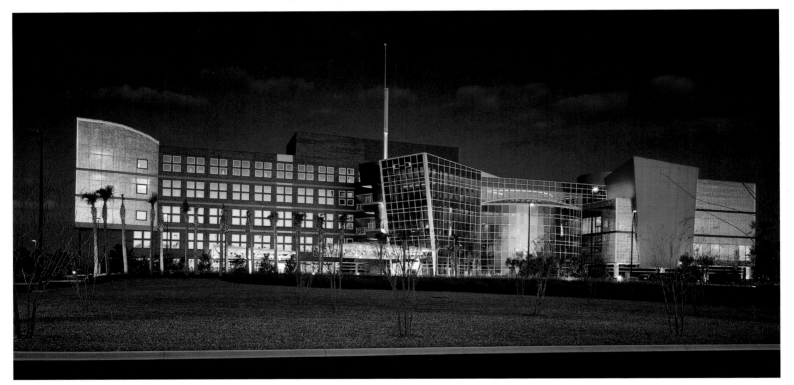

ARCHITECT'S STATEMENT

This new medical center is designed as a "one-stop shopping center" for health care services. It combines a 141-bed acute care hospital with physician suites, health services, and related retail shops. Patients will use the medical center as a source for health promotion and wellness, as well as for rehabilitation from injury and disease. The hospital and physicians work in partnership to provide convenient, efficient health care using emerging technologies and computer link-ups. The center contains more than 50,000 square feet of office space for physicians.

The 9,000-square-foot atrium is surrounded by glass; palm trees and greenery create a feeling of bringing the outdoors in. The atrium hosts a variety of community events, from art shows and children's choir concerts to health fairs and screenings. Registration for hospital services resembles a hotel check-in desk, and most outpatient testing procedures are just a few steps from the registration area.

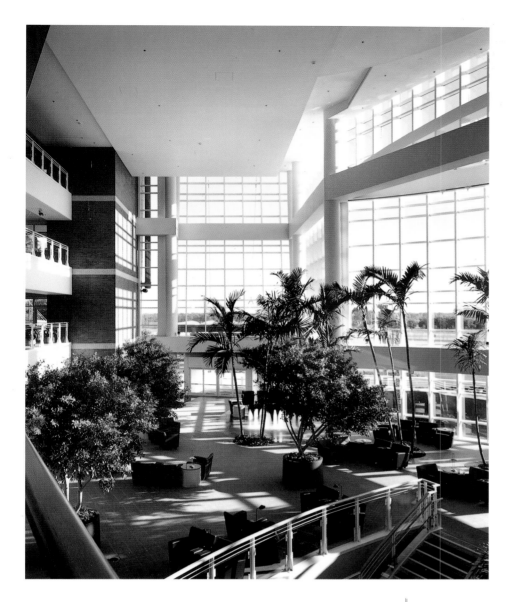

Owner
West Orange Hospital

Data

Type of Facility
Replacement hospital

Context
Hospital-based: 141 beds

Type of Construction
New

Area of Building
260,000 GSF

Cost of Construction
$32,000,000

Cost of Medical Equipment
$5,100,000

Status of Project
Completed February 1993

Credits

Architect
HKS, Inc.
Lincoln Center
5401 W. Kennedy Boulevard,
Suite 1090
Tampa, Florida 33609

Structural Engineer
HKS/Structural
Dallas, Texas

Mechanical Engineer/Electrical Engineer
Smith Seckman Reid, Inc.
Nashville, Tennessee

Landscape Architect
Herbert-Halback, Inc.
Orlando, Florida

Medical Equipment Planner
Mitchell International
Skokie, Illinois

Interior Design
HKS/Designcare
Dallas, Texas

Contractor
The Robins & Morton Corporation
Birmingham, Alabama

Photographer
Michael Lowry
Orlando, Florida

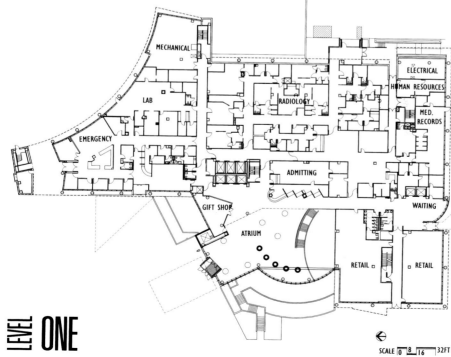

LEVEL ONE

SCALE 0 8 16 32FT

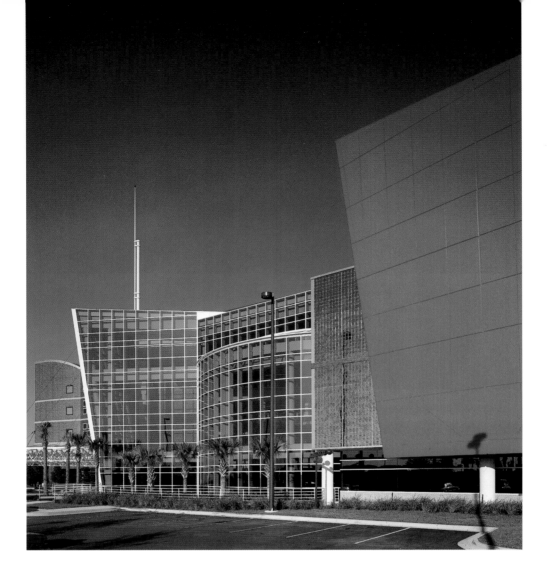

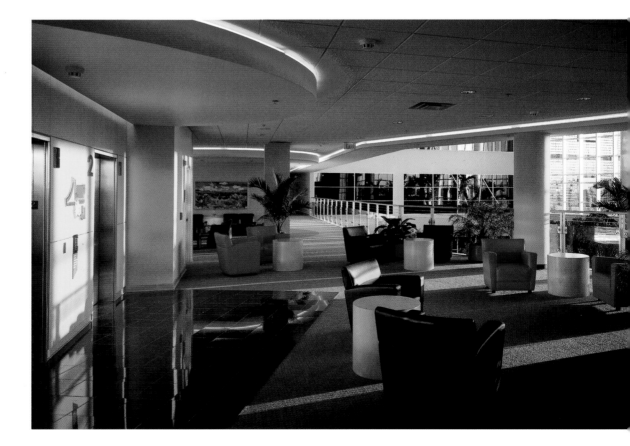

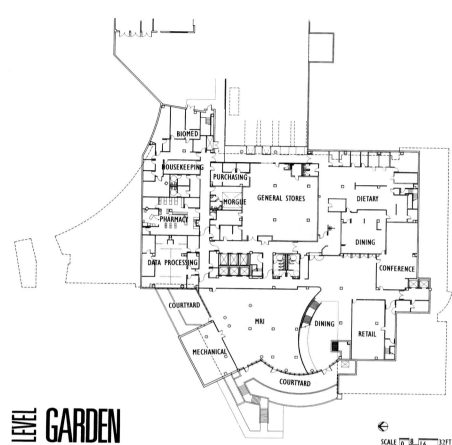

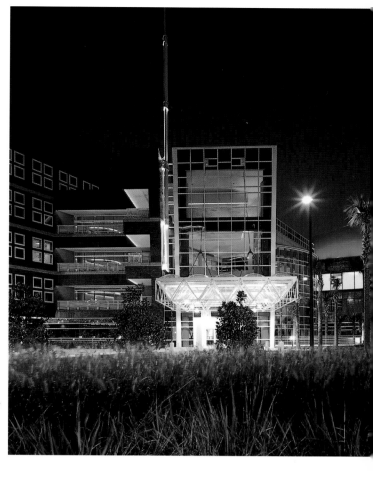

LEVEL GARDEN

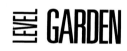

BIOMED

HOUSEKEEPING

PURCHASING

GENERAL STORES

DIETARY

MORGUE

PHARMACY

DINING

DATA PROCESSING

CONFERENCE

COURTYARD

MRI

DINING

RETAIL

MECHANICAL

COURTYARD

SCALE 0 8 16 32FT

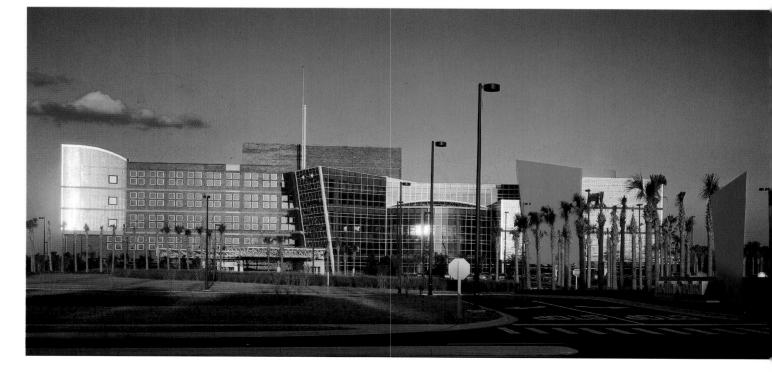

High Desert Medical Center

Los Angeles, California

Citation

This project was considered outstanding among a number of entries that "unbundle" inpatient, outpatient, D & T, and support services. An apparent construction budget of more than $300 per square foot places it at the top of this category as well.

The organization of these elements in this instance simultaneously achieves effective functional relationships, logical expandability, and discrete public access to individual service components. The key to the latter is a site plan that organizes access and parking in ways that make way-finding inevitable, and which creates spaces around and between buildings that are as elegant and serene as the buildings themselves.

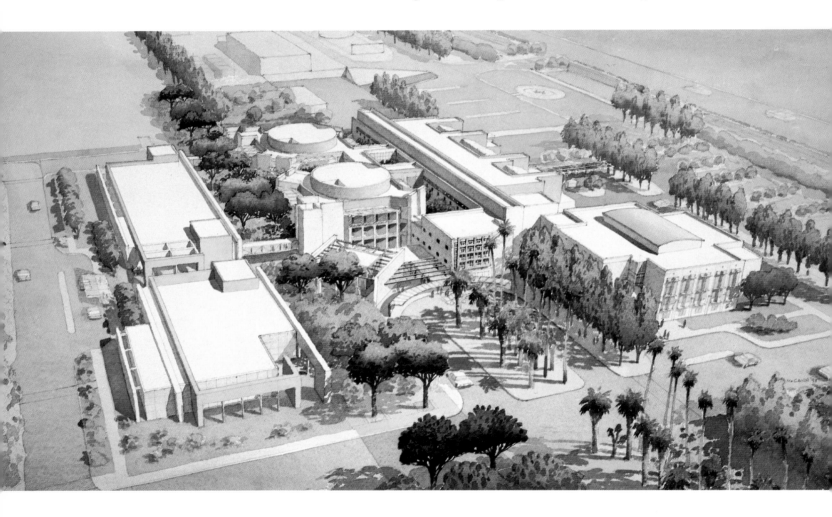

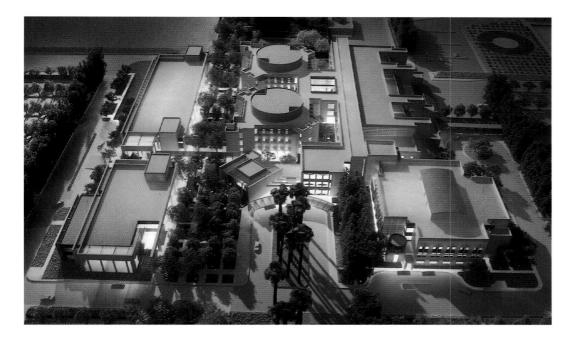

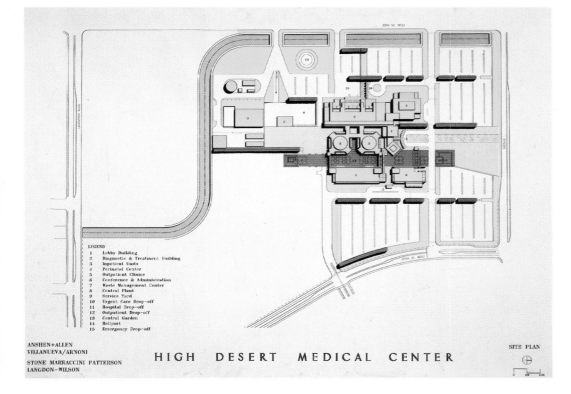

LEGEND
1 Lobby Building
2 Diagnostic & Treatment Building
3 Inpatient Units
4 Perinatal Center
5 Outpatient Clinics
6 Conference & Administration
7 Waste Management Center
8 Central Plant
9 Service Yard
10 Urgent Care Drop-off
11 Hospital Drop-off
12 Outpatient Drop-off
13 Central Garden
14 Heliport
15 Emergency Drop-off

ANSHEN+ALLEN
VILLANUEVA/ARNONI
STONE MARRACCINI PATTERSON
LANGDON—WILSON

HIGH DESERT MEDICAL CENTER

SITE PLAN

ARCHITECT'S STATEMENT

Situated on a broad expanse of desert highland northeast of Los Angeles, the High Desert Medical Center brings inpatient, outpatient, and health education services to a young, expanding community. Interconnected but separate structures in an "unbundled" arrangement house the various services of the medical center, allowing for flexibility and expandability. The north–south axis of the gardens defines the character of the medical center and helps organize and unite its various components. The design makes use of the landscape, both natural and cultivated, to create an environment that encourages healing and rehabilitation.

Owner
County of Los Angeles, Department of Health Services

Data

Type of Facility
Comprehensive medical center

Context
Hospital-based: 200 beds

Type of Construction
New

Area of Building
454,436 GSF

Cost of Construction
$143,000,000

Cost of Medical Equipment
$14,000,000

Status of Project
Estimated date of completion:
June 1999

Credits

Executive Architect
Anshen + Allen Architects, Inc.
5055 Wilshire Boulevard,
Suite 900
Los Angeles, California 90036-4306

Joint Venture Architects
Stone Marraccini Patterson
225 Arizona Avenue
Santa Monica, California 90401

Langdon Wilson
1055 Wilshire Boulevard,
Suite 1500
Los Angeles, California 90017-2449

Villanueva/Arnoni Architects
245 Fischer Avenue, Suite A-3
Costa Mesa, California 92626

Phase I Architect
Lee, Burkhart, Liu
2890 Colorado Avenue
Santa Monica, California 90401

Executive Engineer
Ove Arup & Partners California, Inc.
Los Angeles, California

Structural Engineer
Sinclair & Associates
Los Angeles, California

(credits continue)

Mechanical/Electrical Engineer

T.M.A.D. Engineers, Inc.
Ontario, California

Civil Engineer

The Keith Companies —
North Counties, Inc.
Palmdale, California

Landscape Architect

Pamela Burton & Company
Santa Monica, California

Materials Management and Transportation

Lerch Bates Hospital Group, Inc.
Petaluma, California

Interior Design

Fong and Miyagawa Design
Associates
Los Angeles, California

Cost Estimating

Adamson Associates
Santa Monica, California

Construction Manager

JCM/Hill
Los Angeles, California

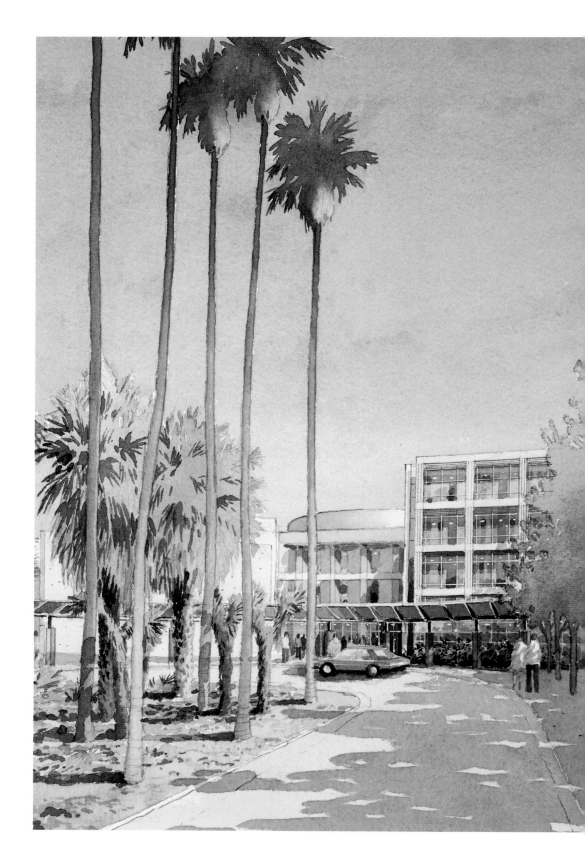

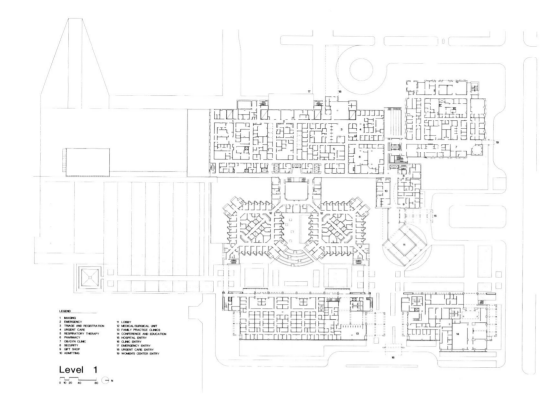

Level 1

0 10 20 40   80   N

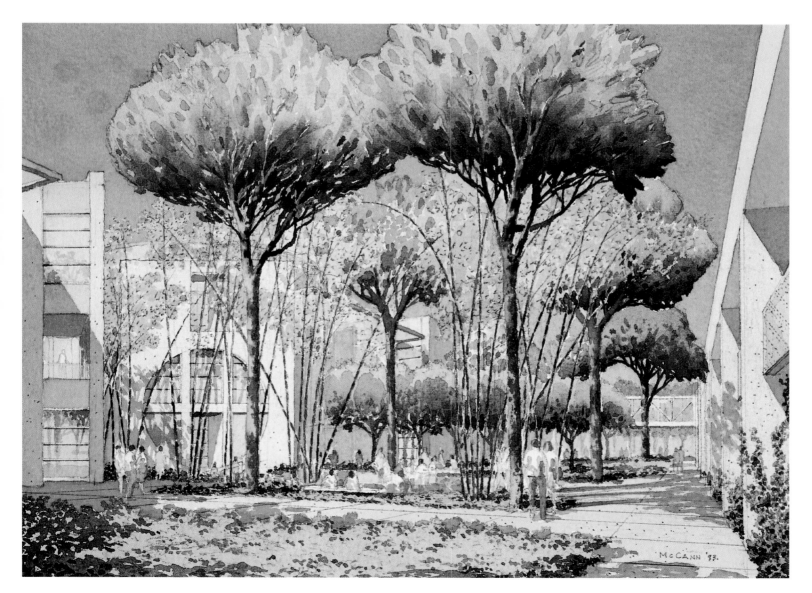

Mary Washington Hospital

Fredericksburg, Virginia

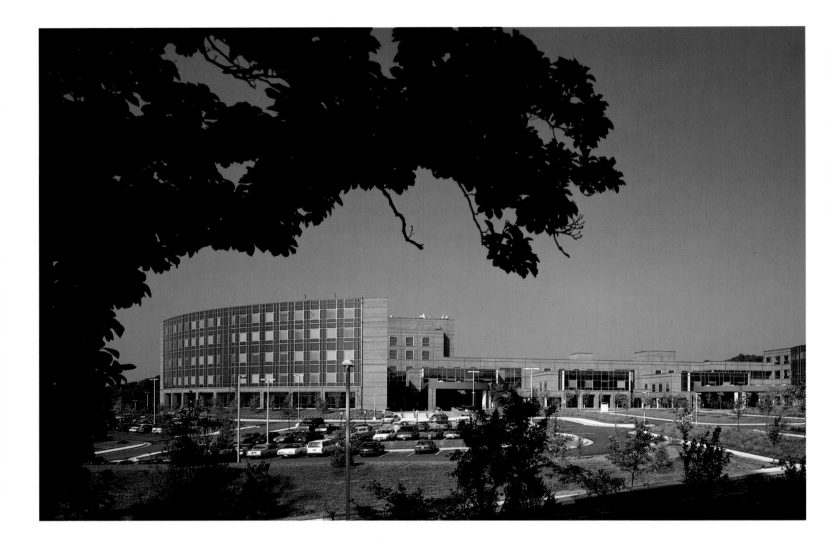

Citation

This project economically accommodates a very large program while creating an easily comprehended and efficient plan, providing for reasonable expansion and change and organizing outpatient and inpatient areas with separate access to diagnostic and treatment care. Access to the hospital and medical office building is clear from Hospital Boulevard to appropriately sized and located parking areas and building entrances.

Building massing, choice of materials and colors, modulation of brick and glass areas, and careful detailing combine to provide a handsome, appropriate enclosure for the various occupancies housed.

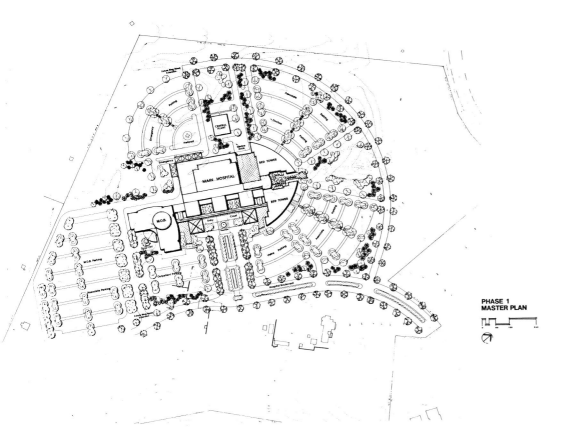

**PHASE 1
MASTER PLAN**

ARCHITECT'S STATEMENT

The building site is a plateau overlooking a small canal and wetlands. All inpatient rooms provide the patients with a panoramic view to the north and east, featuring a dramatic glimpse of the city. When viewed from a distance, the main hospital presents a sleek, engaging, noninstitutional profile. Other components of the hospital were broken down and expressed individually, creating a more human scale. In recognition of the historical era, brick was used to complement and soften the impact of the glass.

The hospital is organized along a public concourse. Departments are attached for easy expansion or relocation. The concourse terminates at the patient care tower, which is also vertically expandable. All bed units were designed to be virtually interchangeable and allow for flexibility in caring for patients at differing levels of need and acuity. As inpatients become more critical, the patient rooms are designed to easily convert to a higher intensity of care. Full capability rooms with built-in features for conversion to critical care are provided.

Owner
Mary Washington Hospital

Data

Type of Facility
Replacement hospital

Context
Hospital-based: 310 beds

Type of Construction
New

Area of Building
438,944 GSF

Cost of Construction
$64,600,000

Cost of Medical Equipment
$9,000,000

Status of Project
Completed July 1993

Credits

Architect
HKS, Inc.
700 N. Pearl Street, Suite 1100
Dallas, Texas 75201

Structural Engineer
HKS/Structural
Dallas, Texas

Mechanical Engineer/Electrical Engineer
Smith Seckman Reid, Inc.
Nashville, Tennessee

Interior Design
HKS/Designcare
Dallas, Texas

Medical Equipment Planner
H.E.L.P. International
Plano, Texas

Food Service Consultants
Mulhauser/McCleary
Associates, Inc.
Dallas, Texas

Contractor
Centex-Rodgers Construction
Company
Nashville, Tennessee

Photographer
Rick Grunbaum
Dallas, Texas

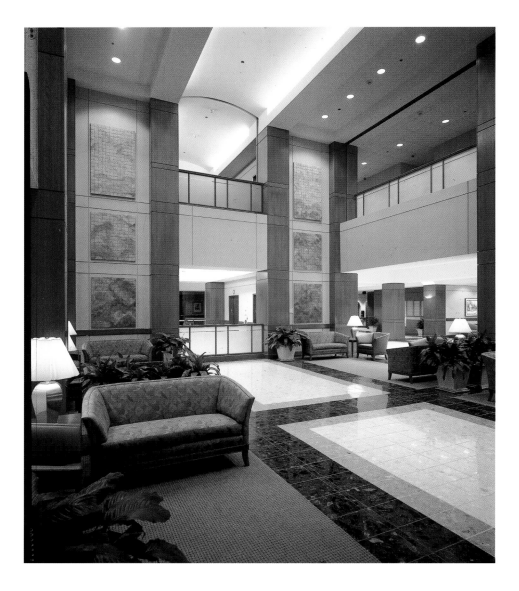

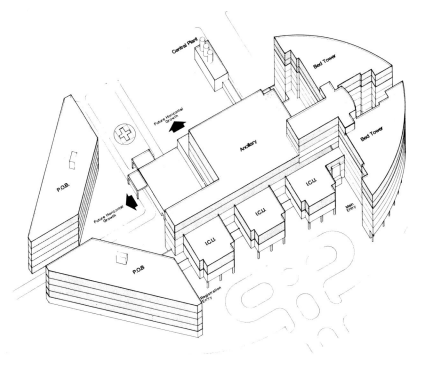

Axonometric

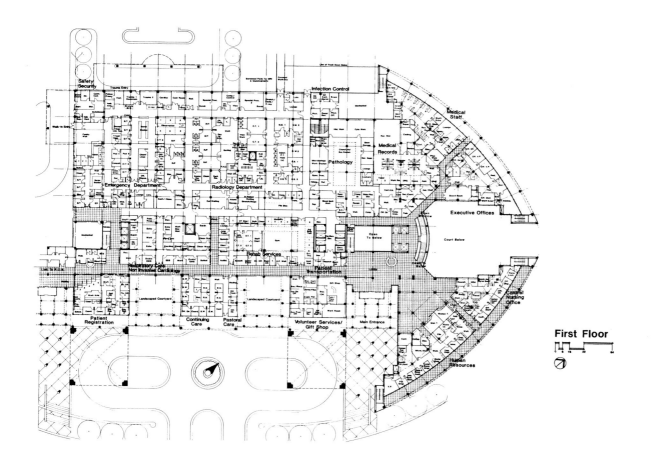

First Floor

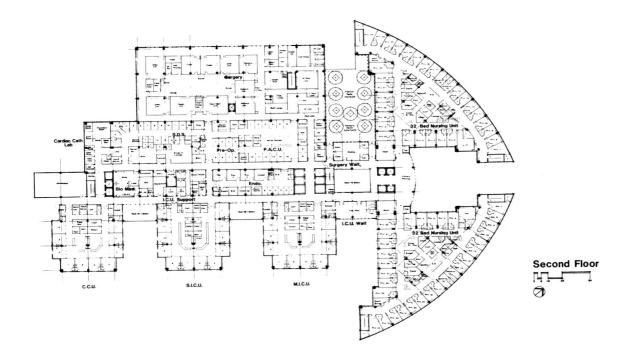

Second Floor

Augusta Medical Center

Fishersville, Virginia

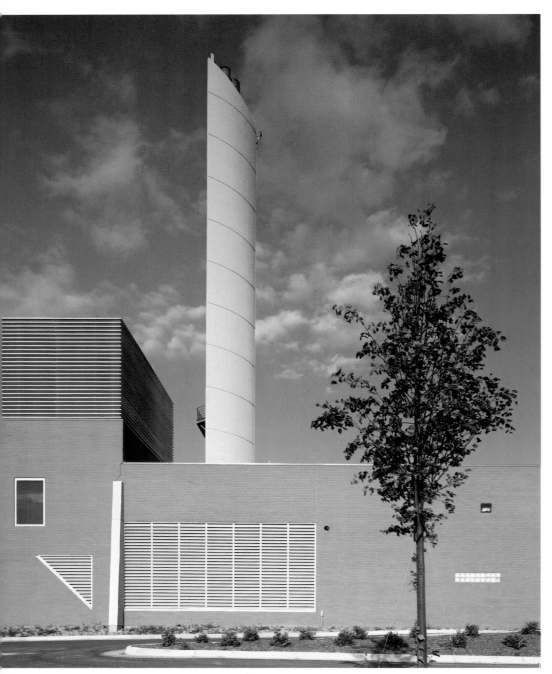

ARCHITECT'S STATEMENT

Two communities decided to pool their resources and build a new hospital to serve their growing needs. This medical center provides state-of-the-art, comprehensive inpatient, outpatient, high-tech ancillary,logistical, and administrative services. Hospital administrators challenged the architect to achieve the site development and building design on a budget of $125 per square foot, with a focus on a design that reduces operating and maintenance costs and improves patient care and staff efficiency.

The design of the medical center combines ideas from human physiology with familiar architectural elements found in the two communities, resulting in an understandable organization of health care and patient services within a technologically sophisticated and flexible environment. A well-defined, dedicated main street circulation system directs outpatients along a corridor of diagnostic services and retail amenities, while a separate circulation system is dedicated to inpatients. Natural light and outdoor views help orient patients, visitors, and staff throughout the facility. Staff efficiency has been improved by reducing travel distances with back-to-back stations and private patient rooms organized in a corrugated corridor pattern.

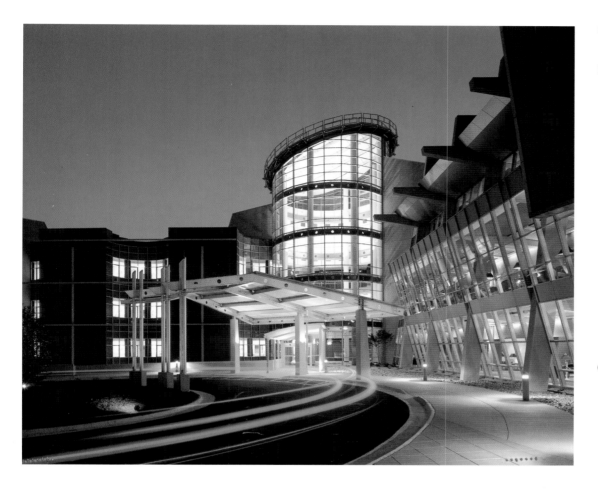

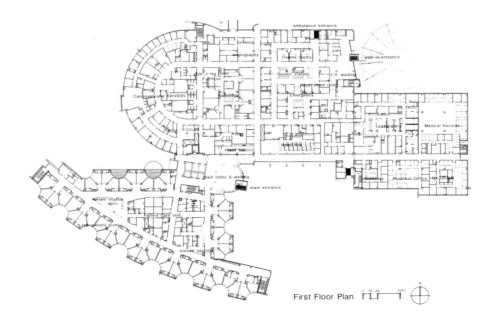

First Floor Plan

Owner
Augusta Hospital Corporation

Data

Type of Facility
Hospital

Context
Hospital-based: 256 beds

Type of Construction
New

Area of Building
389,640 GSF

Cost of Construction
$45,454,403

Cost of Medical Equipment
$6,845,025

Status of Project
Completed August 1994

Credits

Architect
Ellerbe Becket
1875 Connecticut Avenue, N.W.,
Suite 600
Washington, D.C. 20009

Mechanical/Structural/Electrical Engineer
Ellerbe Becket
Washington, D.C.

Civil Engineer
Patton Harris Rust & Associates,
P.C.
Fairfax, Virginia

Programming Consultant
Hamilton/KSA
Fairfax, Virginia

Landscape Architecture
Lee & Liu Associates, Inc.
Washington, D.C.

Food Service Consultants
FOODESIGN Associates, Inc.
Charlotte, North Carolina

Contractor
McCarthy Brothers Company
St. Louis, Missouri

Photographer
Maxwell MacKenzie
Washington, D.C.

Baldwin Park Medical Center

Baldwin Park, California

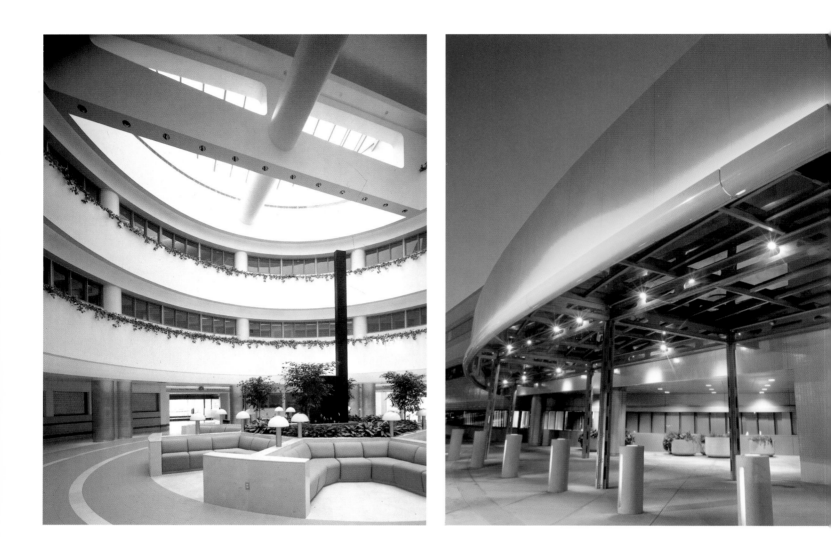

ARCHITECT'S STATEMENT

Baldwin Park Medical Center is a 273-bed acute care facility housed in approximately 850,000 square feet of integrated inpatient/outpatient clinics, surgical suites, and medical office space, including all ancillary spaces required by contemporary health care practice. Hospitality issues affecting patient and staff comfort received primary attention during the design process and resulted in an environment that is conducive to the healing process.

The hospital is situated in a parklike setting with a clear separation between vehicular and pedestrian traffic. Bright yellow canopies clearly identify entry areas. Inside the facility, daylight is used extensively to reduce the institutional feel of the interior. Way-finding is simplified through interior surface articulation, individualized departmental color schemes, and specially commissioned artwork.

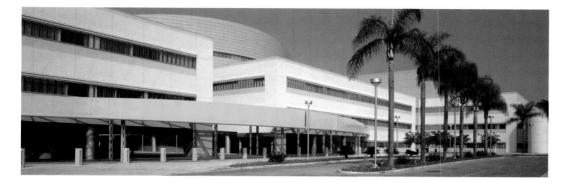

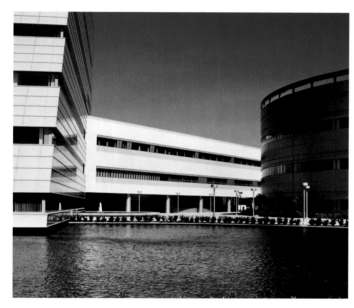

BASEMENT PLAN

1. EDUCATION & TRAINING
2. IN-PATIENT PHARMACY
3. HVAC
4. SHELL-IN
5. FOOD SERVICE
6. QUALITY ASSURANCE
7. CANCER REGISTRY
8. MORGUE
9. MATERIALS MANAGEMENT
10. LINEN
11. CLEAN DOCK
12. SOILED DOCK
13. PLANT OPERATIONS & EQUIPMENT
14. OUTPATIENT RECORDS
15. INFORMATION SERVICES
16. CENTRAL PROCESSING
17. HOSPITAL RECORDS
18. ENVIRONMENTAL SERVICES
19. STAFF
20. MEDICAL OFFICE BUILDING ABOVE

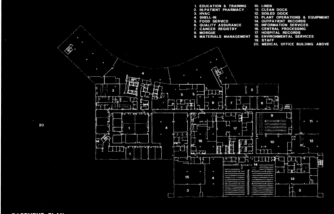

Owner
Kaiser Foundation Hospitals

Data
Type of Facility
Acute care medical center

Context
Hospital-based: 273 beds

Type of Construction
New

Area of Building
849,000 GSF

Cost of Construction
Estimated: $163,100,000

Cost of Medical Equipment
Estimated: $52,200,000

Status of Project
Completed November 1994

Credits
Architect
HMC GROUP, Inc.
3270 Inland Empire Boulevard
Ontario, California

Consulting Architect
Arthur Erickson Associates
125 North Robertson Boulevard
Los Angeles, California 90048

Structural Engineer
Brandow and Johnston Associates
Los Angeles, California

Mechanical Engineer
J.L. Hengstler, Inc.
Glendale, California

Electrical Engineer
Sampson, Randall, and Press, Inc.
Los Angeles, California

Civil Engineer
JHH Consultants
Irvine, California

Cogeneration Consultant
Brown and Caldwel
Pasadena, California

Food Service Consultant
DEWCO
Whittier, California

Traffic Impact Consultants
Donald Frischer & Associates
Van Nuys, California

Graphics Consultant
Follis Design
Pasadena, California

Interior Design
HMC GROUP Interiors Division
Ontario, California

Parking Consultants
International Parking Design, Inc.
Costa Mesa, California

Radiology Planning Consultant
James Staublin Planning
and Design
Westlake Village, California

Art Consultant
Joanna Burke Associates
Venice, California

*Materials Management/Vertical
Transportation Consultant*
Lerch Bates Hospital Group, Inc.
Petaluma, California

Landscape Architect
Randolph Hlubik Associates, Inc.
Riverside, California

Fire Protection Consultant
Rolf Jenson and Associates, Inc.
Concord, California

Contractor Identification
McCarthy Western Constructors
Irvine, California

Photographer
Fred Licht Studios
North Hollywood, California

Baton Rouge General Health Center

Baton Rouge, Louisiana

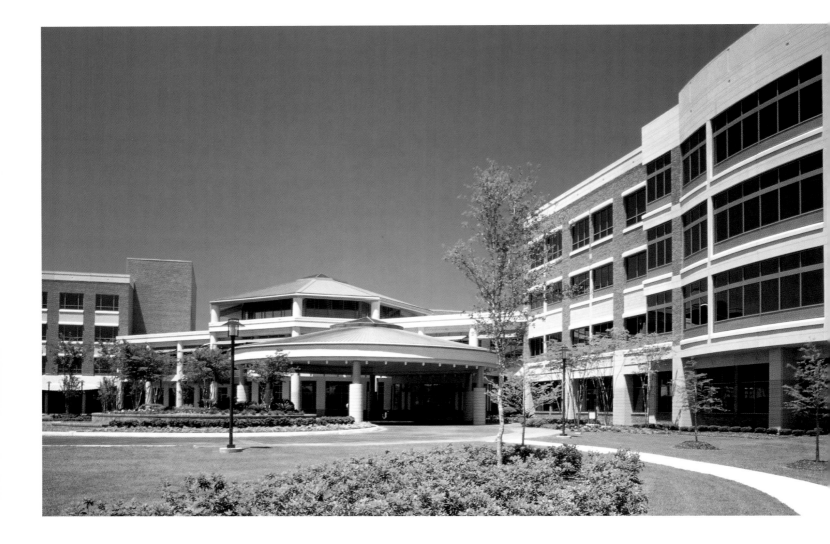

The image, comfort, and convenience of hospitality amenities characterize this new patient-oriented facility. As the core facility of a planned medical campus, the Baton Rouge General Health Center comprises a four-story, 90-bed inpatient wing, a central two-story outpatient health center, and a four-story medical office building.

Multiple entry points are marked with distinctive metal roof canopies showing main public drop-offs.

Extensive use is made of daylight in the interior, with circulation oriented toward a central atrium and landscaped plaza that provide access to the facility's main departments.

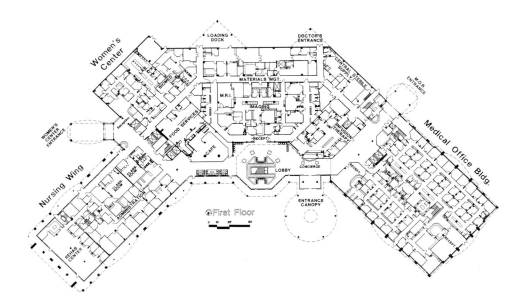

First Floor

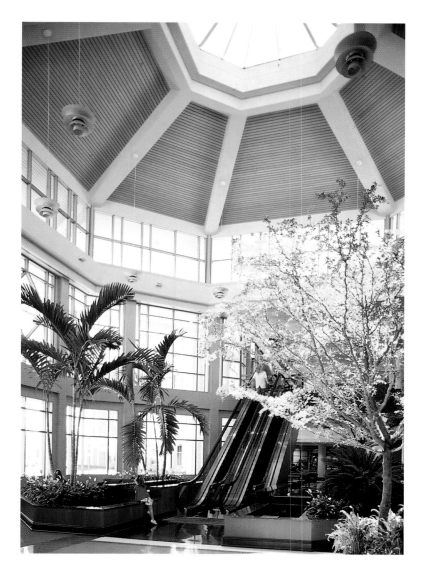

O w n e r
General Health System

D a t a
Type of Facility
Hospital/medical office building

Context
Hospital-based: 90 beds

Type of Construction
New

Area of Building
244,000 GSF

Cost of Construction
$22,600,000

Cost of Medical Equipment
$6,400,000

Status of Project
Completed October 1994

C r e d i t s
Architect
Washer, Hill & Lipscomb Architects
1744 Oakdale Drive
Baton Rouge, Louisiana 70810

Structural Engineer
Ragland Aderman & Associates
Baton Rouge, Louisiana

Mechanical Engineer
Mayers & Associates
Baton Rouge, Louisiana

Electrical Engineer
Calongne & Associates
Baton Rouge, Louisiana

Landscape Architect
Henslee-Cox Landscape Architects
Baton Rouge, Louisiana

Interior Design
Leslie Herpin Interior Design
Baton Rouge, Louisiana

Lighting Design
Paulette Hebert Lighting Consultant
Baton Rouge, Louisiana

Contractor
Milton J. Womack Construction
Co., Inc.
Baton Rouge, Louisiana

Photographer
Rex Cabaniss
Baton Rouge, Louisiana

Clinical Improvement Addition
Richard Roudebush Veterans Affairs Medical Center

Indianapolis, Indiana

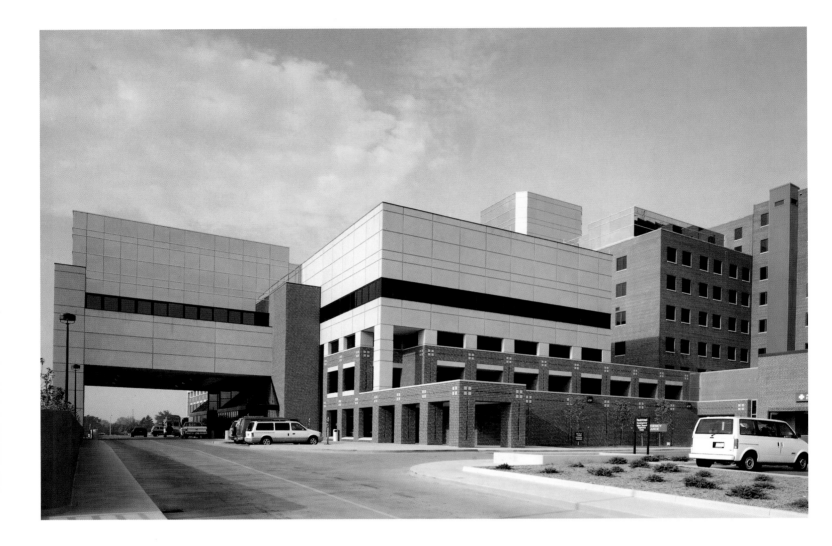

ARCHITECT'S STATEMENT

The Clinical Improvement Addition to the Richard L. Roudebush Veterans Affairs Medical Center is one of two additions to the Indianapolis campuses. The West Tenth Street campus is next to the Indiana University Medical Center and comprises an assortment of additions. This new addition replaces all high-technology areas of the hospital and allows the hospital to consolidate all its ambulatory care programs.

The design was intended to expand on the existing building materials using the brick-and-stone color patterns and masonry window piers to provide relief from the linear appearance of the building facade. The mirrored curtain wall elevator tower was used as a transition between the new and existing buildings. The main entrance to the new building was designed to be monumental in appearance and to signify the primary access point into the building for patients and visitors. An underground parking structure was included in the design to offset the loss of surface parking caused by the new building footprint.

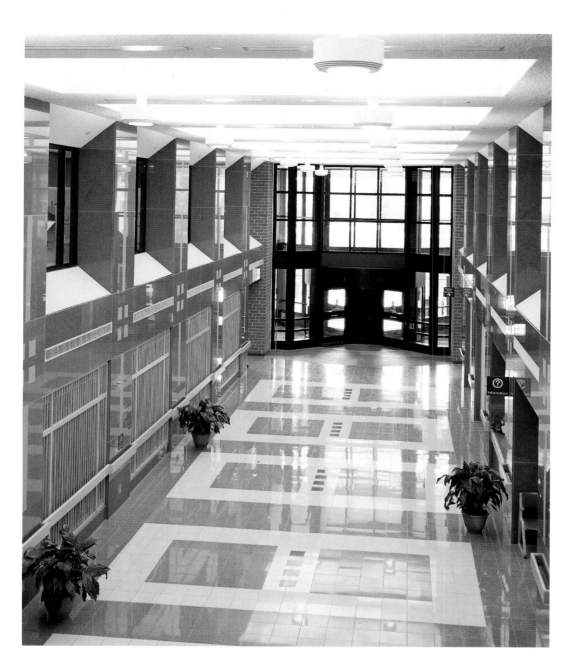

Owner
U.S. Department of Veterans Affairs

Data

Type of Facility
Hospital addition

Context
Hospital-based

Type of Construction
New

Area of Building
501,000 GSF

Cost of Construction
$42,000,000

Cost of Medical Equipment
$4,000,000

Status of Project
Completed October 1994

Credits

Architect
BSA Design
6810 North Shadeland Avenue
Indianapolis, Indiana 46220

Structural/Mechanical/Electrical Engineer
BSA Design
Indianapolis, Indiana

Food Facilities Equipment
Vondran & Associates
Fort Wayne, Indiana

Vertical Transportation
Syska & Hennessy
San Francisco, California

Cost Estimating
Beach, McCarthy & Donaldson Associates
Martinez, California

Contractor
Centex Bateson
Dallas, Texas

Photographer
Mardan Photography
Indianapolis, Indiana

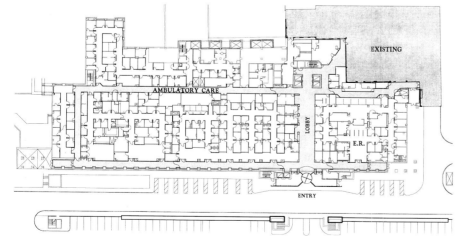

SITE PLAN

0 8 16 32   NORTH

Composite Medical Facility, 3rd Medical Center

Elmendorf Air Force Base, Anchorage, Alaska

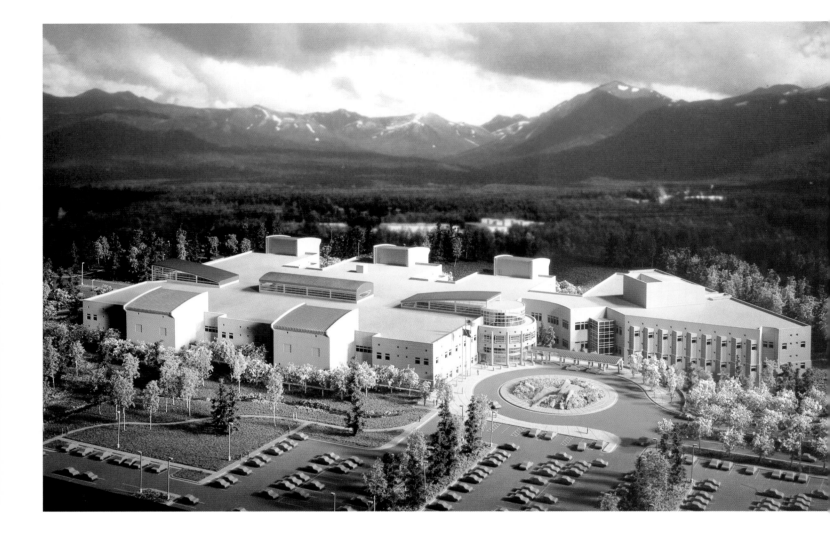

ARCHITECT'S STATEMENT

The project consolidates all services into a single, state-of-the-art medical facility, the largest in Alaska. The building's scale is manipulated through massing to achieve pedestrian-level texture and detail. As a medical facility in an area prone to strong earthquakes, the building not only must withstand such seismic activity but remain fully operational in its aftermath. The design includes a square structural grid, precast-concrete building skin that moves with seismic force, a safe but flexible attachment system, and backups for all utility systems.

The facility is organized around a medical mall that contains clinic waiting areas and public support functions, and simplifies user orientation and access. Departments are planned in three zones: eight-hour clinical uses, 24-hour ancillary departments, and nursing units. The most active spaces are on the first floor; other specialty departments are on the second. An Integrated Building System allows the building to adapt easily to planning changes. For example, outboard mechanical and electrical utility pods and a walk-on service deck between floors allow maintenance and service to occur quickly, cost-effectively, and with minimal disruption. Construction time is reduced since multiple trades can work simultaneously.

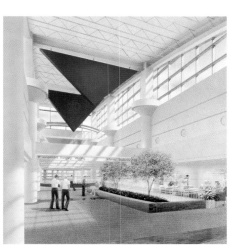

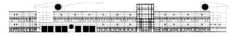

NORTH ELEVATION

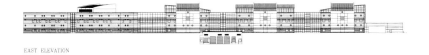

EAST ELEVATION

SOUTH ELEVATION

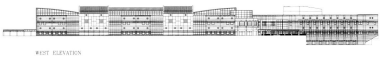

WEST ELEVATION

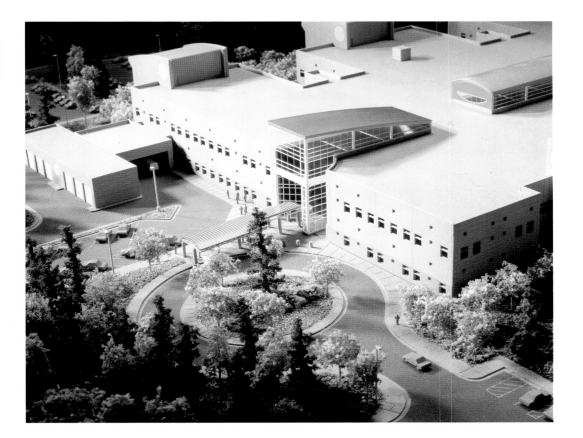

Owner
United States Air Force

Data

Type of Facility
Comprehensive health care facility

Context
Hospital-based: 110 beds

Type of Construction
New

Area of Building
434,258 GSF

Cost of Construction
Bid estimate: $131,000,000

Cost of Medical Equipment
Bid estimate: $5,446,000

Status of Project
Estimated date of completion:
September 1998

Credits

Architect
Anderson DeBartolo Pan
2480 N. Arcadia Avenue
Tucson, Arizona 85712

Associate Architect
Maynard & Partch
4007 Old Seward Highway,
Suite 800
Anchorage, Alaska 99503

Design / Construction Agent
U.S. Army Corps of Engineers
Washington, D.C.

*Structural / Mechanical / Electrical
Engineer*
Anderson DeBartolo Pan
Tucson, Arizona

Associate Structural Engineer
Loftus & Daily, Inc.
Minneapolis, Minnesota

*Associate Mechanical / Electrical / Fire
Engineer*
Alaska Engineering Consultants, Inc.
Anchorage, Alaska

Civil and Landscape Engineers
DOWL Engineers, Inc.
Anchorage, Alaska (civil)
Redmond, Washington (landscape)

Contractor
M.A. Mortenson
Minneapolis, Minnesota

Photographer
Balfour Walker
Tucson, Arizona

Crow/Northern Cheyenne Indian Health Service Hospital

Crow Agency, Montana

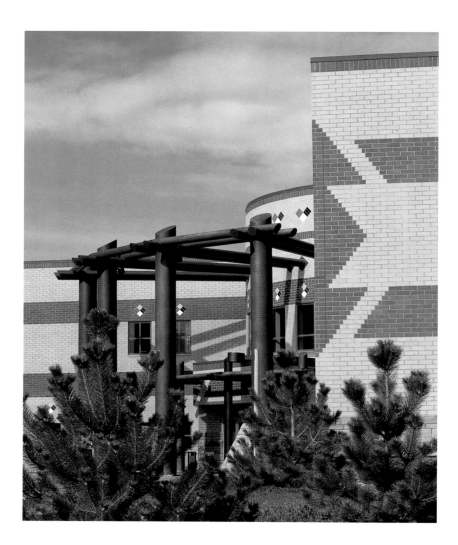

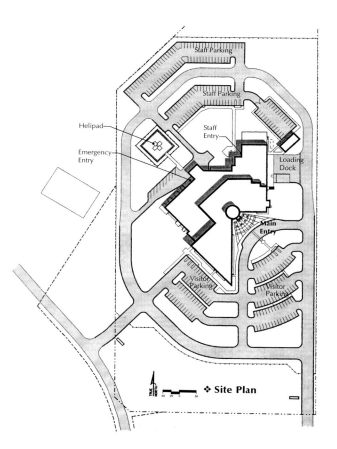

❖ **Site Plan**

ARCHITECT'S STATEMENT

The Crow/Northern Cheyenne Indian Health Service Hospital, located in Crow Agency, Montana, serves approximately 12,500 Native Americans in south-central Montana. The Indian Health Service (IHS) is a federal component that delivers health care to the Crow and Northern Cheyenne Indian tribes.

The program requirements established by the IHS called for a facility with 24 inpatient beds, surgery/delivery capability, and extensive ambulatory services. The unique challenge of this project was to design a large, modern health care facility that assembled building materials, shapes, and colors to reflect the cultures of two Indian tribes that historically had been enemies. As one user stated early in design, "the building could serve as a bridge between the two tribes."

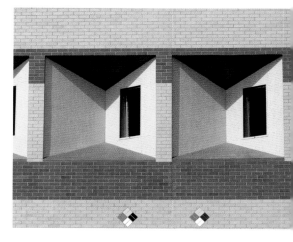

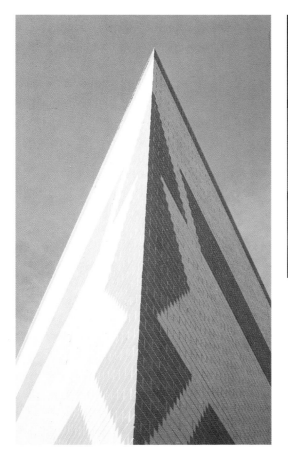

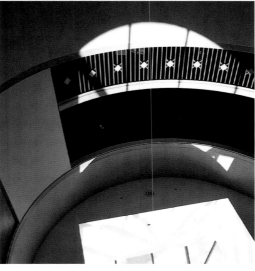

O w n e r

Public Health Service, Indian
Health Service

D a t a

Type of Facility

Comprehensive facility, primarily
outpatient services

Context

Hospital-based: 24 beds

Type of Construction

New

Area of Building

95,515 GSF

Cost of Construction

$14,850,000

Cost of Medical Equipment

$3,447,000

Status of Project

Completed March 1995

C r e d i t s

Architect

CTA Architects Engineers
1500 Poly Drive
Billings, Montana 59102

Medical Planning Consultant

Medical Planning Associates
1601 Rambla Pacifico
Malibu, California 90265

*Structural / Mechanical / Electrical
Engineer*

CTA Architects Engineers
Billings, Montana

Civil Engineer

Engineering, Inc.
Billings, Montana

Federal Contract / Project Management

Public Health Service
Office of Engineering Services,
Region X
Seattle, Washington

Cultural Consultant

Little Big Horn Community College
Crow Agency, Montana

Food Service Design

Thomas Ricca Associates
Englewood, Colorado

Contractor

Swank Enterprises
Valier, Montana

Photographer

High Plains Production, Inc.
Billings, Montana

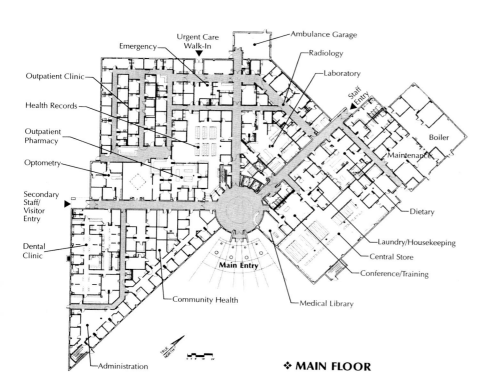

❖ **MAIN FLOOR**

Cullman Regional Medical Center

Cullman, Alabama

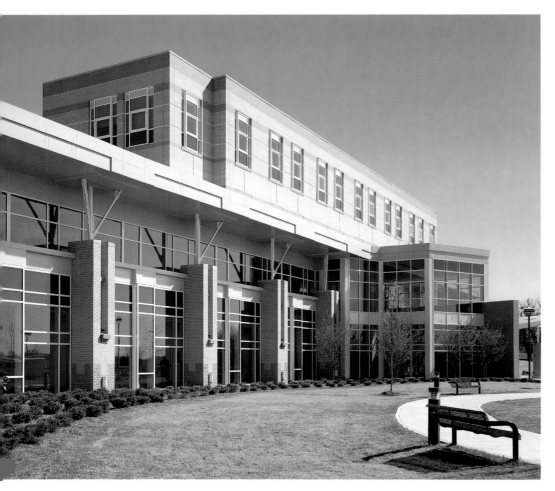

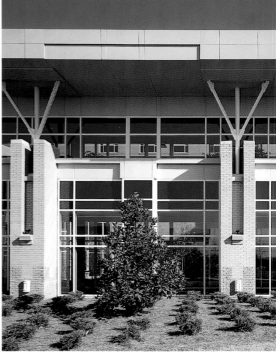

A R C H I T E C T ' S   S T A T E M E N T

This total replacement of an obsolete hospital structure responds to increased demand for emergency and outpatient services and the need to downsize inpatient nursing units. The overall planning/design concept is based on the goals of providing user convenience and friendliness, flexibility for future change, open-ended paths for future growth, and building efficiency through the grouping of similar functions. Separate entrances to patient drop-off, outpatient service, and the emergency room provide easy patient and visitor access. The design emphasizes the natural healing qualities of the rural landscape. Abundant glass gives the building a transparent quality and allows pleasant views from many perspectives.

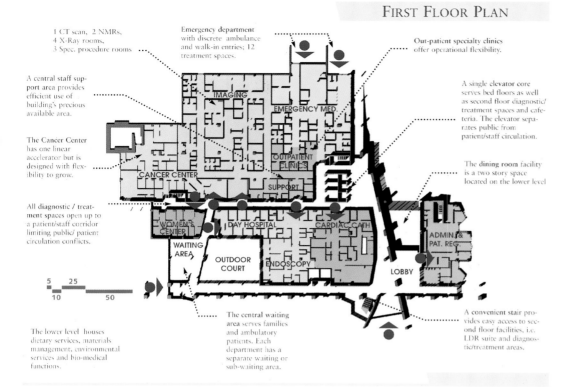

1 CT scan, 2 NMRs, 4 X-Ray rooms, 3 Spec. procedure rooms

Emergency department with discrete ambulance and walk-in entries; 12 treatment spaces.

Out-patient specialty clinics offer operational flexibility.

A central staff support area provides efficient use of building's precious available area.

A single elevator core serves bed floors as well as second floor diagnostic/treatment spaces and cafeteria. The elevator separates public from patient/staff circulation.

The Cancer Center has one linear accelerator but is designed with flexibility to grow.

The dining room facility is a two story space located on the lower level

All diagnostic / treatment spaces open up to a patient/staff corridor limiting public/ patient circulation conflicts.

The lower level houses dietary services, materials management, environmental services and bio-medical functions.

The central waiting area serves families and ambulatory patients. Each department has a separate waiting or sub-waiting area.

A convenient stair provides easy access to second floor facilities, i.e. LDR suite and diagnostic/treatment areas.

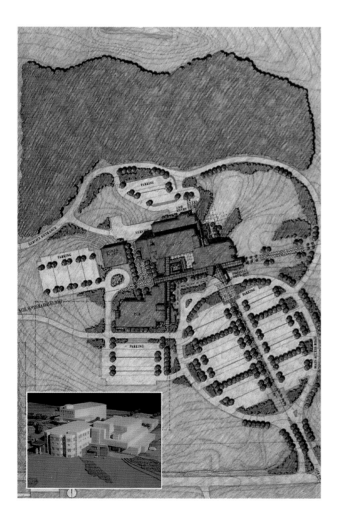

Owner

Cullman Regional Medical Center— an affiliate hospital of Baptist Health System

Data

Type of Facility
Hospital replacement

Context
Hospital-based: 115 beds

Type of Construction
New

Area of Building
218,000 GSF

Cost of Construction
$22,954,800

Cost of Medical Equipment
$7,752,000

Status of Project
Completed January 1995

Credits

Architect
TRO/The Ritchie Organization
115 Twenty-First Street North
Birmingham, Alabama

Structural Engineer
Marlin, Bridges & Associates, Inc., Structural Engineers
Birmingham, Alabama

Mechanical Engineer
Miller & Weaver, Inc.
Birmingham, Alabama

Electrical Engineer
Ray Engineering Group
Birmingham, Alabama

Civil Engineer
St. John & Associates
Cullman, Alabama

Landscape Architect
Nimrod Long & Associates
Birmingham, Alabama

Hospital Materials Management/Transportation
Lerch Bates Hospital Group, Inc.
Timonium, Maryland

Equipment Planning
The Meyer Group
Orlando, Florida

Interior Design
CLJ Associates
Birmingham, Alabama

Traffic and Planning Consultant
Gorove/Slade Associates, Inc.
Birmingham, Alabama

Contractor
Robins & Morton/Eidsen— A Joint Venture
Birmingham, Alabama

Photographers
Timothy Hursley
Little Rock, Arkansas
Randy Lovoy
Birmingham, Alabama

Diagnostic Services Building, St. Francis Regional Medical Center

Wichita, Kansa

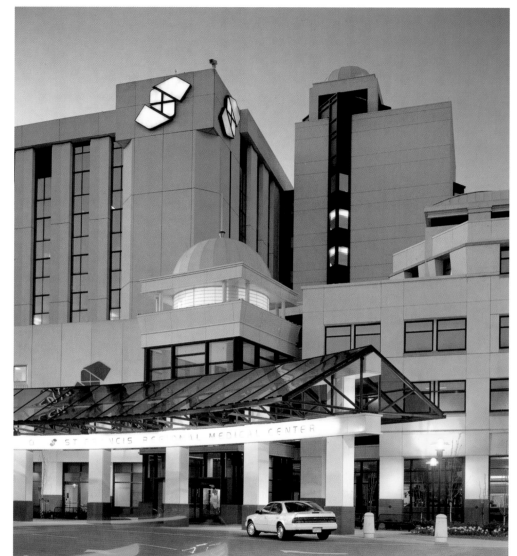

ARCHITECT'S STATEMENT

In an effort to increase market share, this regional medical center undertook a $35 million expansion and renovation project aimed at enhancing its image and improving patient access to services, while updating antiquated diagnostic imaging, laboratory and cardiology services. The five-level addition is sandwiched between a new 750-car garage, an existing nursing tower, and an existing MRI facility. The expansion includes a new main entrance, which is punctuated by an internally illuminated dome resting on top of a new, eight-story elevator tower. The domed tower has become an area landmark that, when illuminated, is visible for miles.

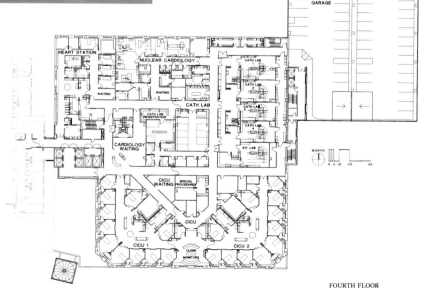

FOURTH FLOOR

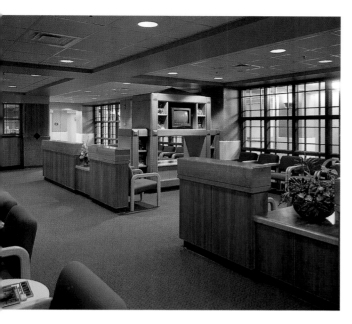

Owner
St. Francis Regional Medical Center

Data

Type of Facility
Inpatient/outpatient diagnostic services

Context
Hospital-based: 20 critical intensive care unit beds

Type of Construction
New and renovation

Area of Building
269,550 GSF (252,575 new; 16,975 renovation)

Cost of Construction
$34,012,650
($33,065,600 new; $947,050 renovation)

Cost of Medical Equipment
$19,433,000

Status of Project
Completed April 1993

Credits

Architect
HNTB Corporation
1201 Walnut, Suite 700
Kansas City, Missouri 64106

Structural Engineer
HNTB Corporation
Kansas City, Missouri

Mechanical/Electrical Engineer
Massaglia Neustrom Bredson, Inc.
Kansas City, Missouri

Civil Engineer
Professional Engineering Corporation
Wichita, Kansas

Landscape Architect
HNTB Corporation
Kansas City, Missouri

Interior Architect
HNTB Corporation
Kansas City, Missouri

Contractor
Dondlinger & Sons Construction Co., Inc.
Wichita, Kansas

Photographer
Mike Sinclair
Sinclair/Reinsch
Kansas City, Missouri

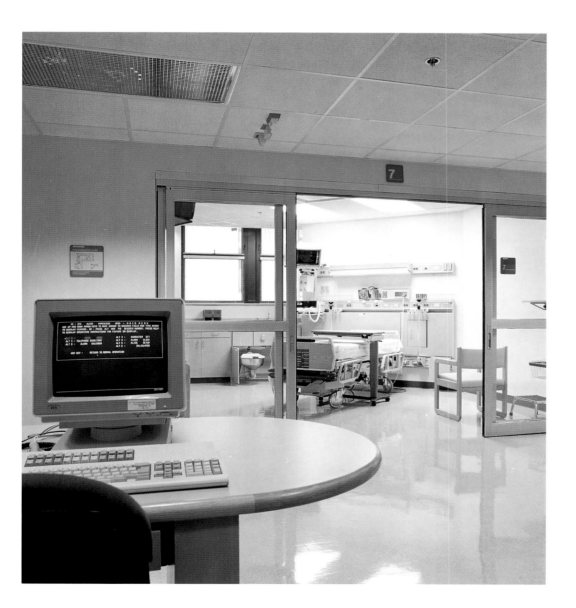

Federal Medical Center

Butner, North Carolina

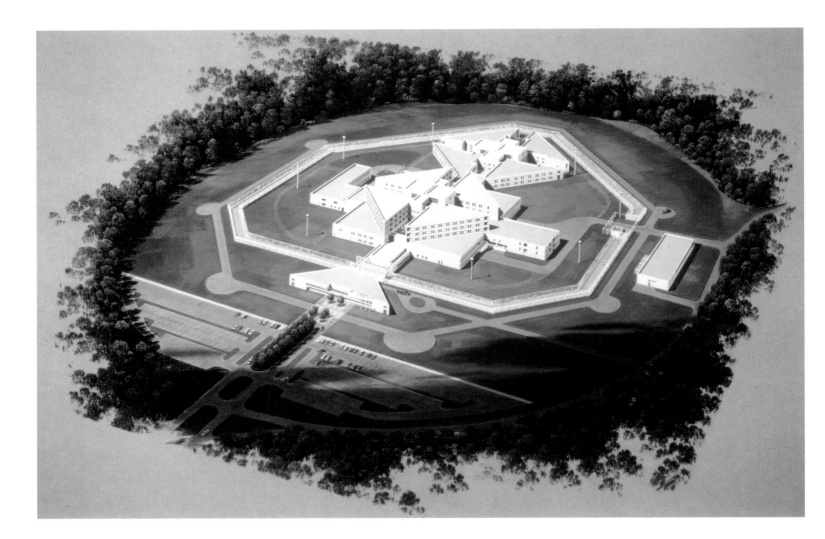

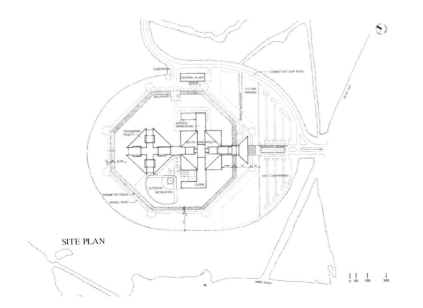

SITE PLAN

The Federal Medical Center (FMC) at Butner, North Carolina, will serve as a prototype program for future facilities in the Federal Bureau of Prisons system. The medical center will be located within the existing Butner complex.

The FMC provides acute medical, surgical, and psychiatric services for both male and female offenders. The FMC will be an administrative facility capable of handling patients of all security levels. High-security patient rooms will be distributed throughout the medical, surgical, and psychiatric units for the housing of high-security inmates.

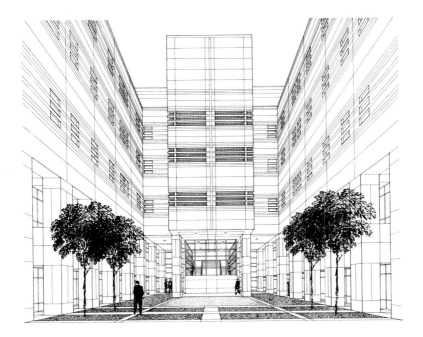

COURTYARD

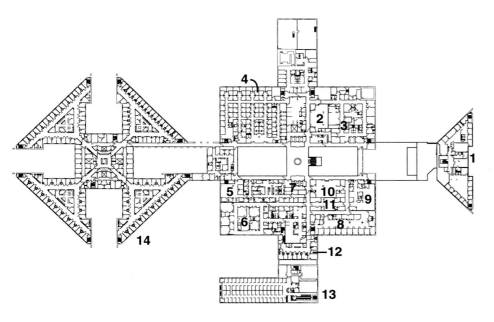

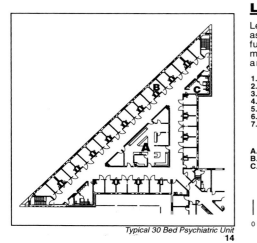

Typical 30 Bed Psychiatric Unit
14

A. Central Nursing Station
B. Typical Patient Room
C. Group Shower / Toilets

0	100	N	

Level 2   FMC

Level **2** includes diagnostic / treatment facilities as well as four 30 bed psychiatric units. Other functions include administration, cadre and mechanical. Separate corridors for staff / patients and visitors overlook the courtyards.

1.	Administration	**8.**	Critical Care
2.	Medical Records	**9.**	Dialysis
3.	Radiology	**10.**	Pharmacy
4.	Ambulatory Care	**11.**	Bio-Medical
5.	Dental	**12.**	Witness Security
6.	Surgery	**13.**	Cadre
7.	Laboratory	**14.**	Psychiatric

Owner

U.S. Department of Justice, Federal Bureau of Prisons

Data

Type of Facility

Comprehensive acute health care and inpatient psychiatric care, plus hospital support inmate population (Cadre)

Context

Hospital-based: 513 beds

Type of Construction

New

Area of Building

632,000 GSF

Cost of Construction

Bid estimate: $67,571,811

Cost of Medical Equipment

Bid estimate: $8,533,635

Status of Project

Estimated completion date: December 1996

Credits

Architect

Odell Associates Inc.
129 West Trade Street
Charlotte, North Carolina 28202

Executive Architect

Middleton, McMillan, Architects
227 West Trade Street
Charlotte, North Carolina 28202

Structural / Mechanical / Electrical Engineer

Odell Associates Inc.
Charlotte, North Carolina

Security Consultant

Buford Goff & Associates
Columbia, South Carolina

Food Service Consultant

Cini-Little International, Inc.
Rockville, Maryland

Equipment Consultant

Facilities Development, Inc.
Phoenix, Arizona

Contractor

Blake Construction Co., Inc.
Washington, D.C.

FHP Medical Campus

Salt Lake City, Utah

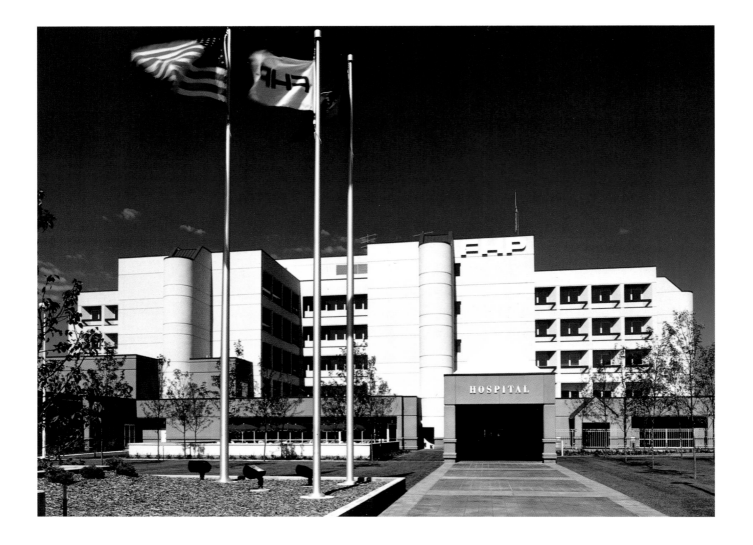

ARCHITECT'S STATEMENT

Until recently, Utah's medical architecture lacked leadership to bring the market into the new, patient-focused, whole-healing approach to design. The new FHP Campus is the first health facility in Utah to be designed with these principles as its focus. Visitors and patients often remark that the environment feels more like a hotel or resort with its open, daylit interiors finished with subdued soft colors and textures. Fine art is displayed throughout to support the healing process. Views and access to the courtyard, landscaped grounds, and the mountain valley support the therapeutic benefits of the interior design. Campus and building circulation is clean and direct. The design accommodates expansion and technology upgrades.

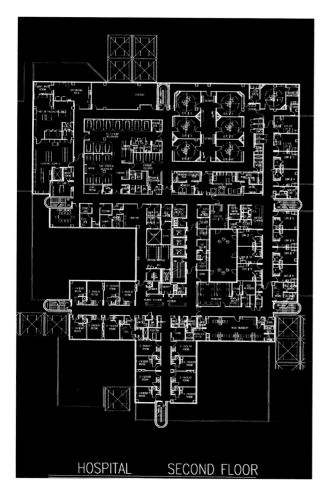

HOSPITAL   SECOND FLOOR

Owner
  FHP, Inc.

Data
  Type of Facility
    Medical campus: hospital, specialty
    center, senior center, hospital
    services, central plant*Context*

    Hospital-based: 201 beds

  Type of Construction
    New

  Area of Buildings
    334,000 GSF

Cost of Construction
  $32,398,531

Cost of Medical Equipment
  $19,518,084

Status of Project
  Completed July 1993

Credits
  Architect
    Valentiner Crane Brunjes Onyon
    Architects
    524 South 600 East
    Salt Lake City, Utah 84102

  Associate Architect
    Dan L. Rowland Architects
    & Associates, Inc.
    6437 East Yosemite
    Orange, California 92667

  Structural Engineer
    Bsumek Mu & Associates
    Salt Lake City, Utah

  Mechanical Engineer
    Van Boerum & Frank Associates
    Salt Lake City, Utah

  Electrical Engineer
    BNA Associates
    Salt Lake City, Utah

  Civil Engineer
    Eckhoff, Watson & Preator
    Salt Lake City, Utah

  Landscape Architect
    MGB&A
    Salt Lake City, Utah

  Interior Design
    BranchWest
    Newport Beach, California

  Contractor
    Big 'D' Construction
    Ogden, Utah

  Photographer
    Scott Zimmerman
    Park City, Utah

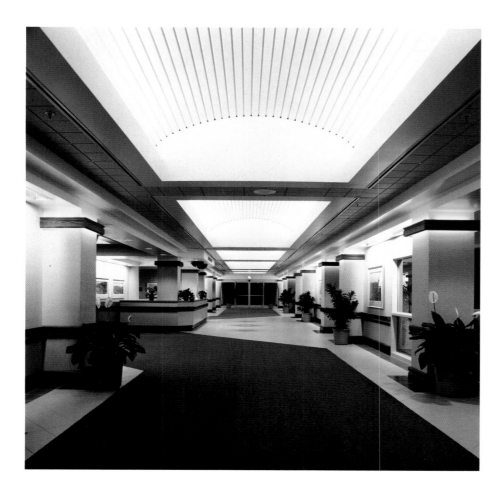

The Homer Gudelsky Building
University of Maryland Medical System

Baltimore, Maryland

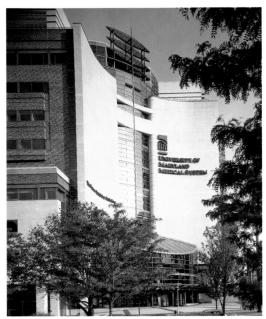

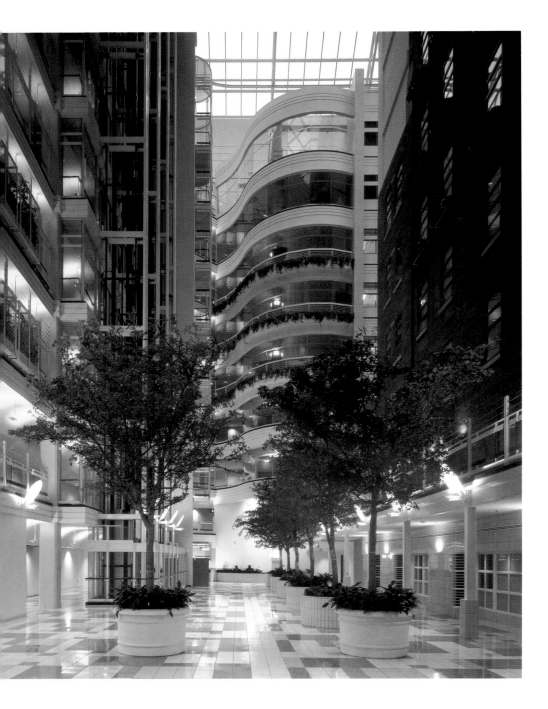

ARCHITECT'S STATMENT

Located on a prominent site in downtown Baltimore, this new addition has an L-shaped plan and is pulled away from the existing building. Between the buildings is an atrium with a glazed roof, part of a major circulation spine and an important orientation area for visitors. Facilities include radiation oncology, nuclear medicine, an ambulatory surgery suite, and administrative services; as well as intensive care units, step-down units, and general care units for cancer treatment, neurology and neurosurgery, cardiac care, cardiothoracic surgery, and transplant surgery.

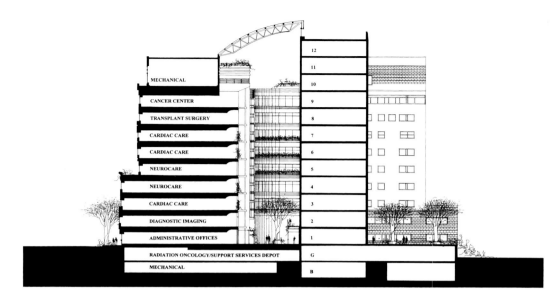

MECHANICAL	12
	11
	10
CANCER CENTER	9
TRANSPLANT SURGERY	8
CARDIAC CARE	7
CARDIAC CARE	6
NEUROCARE	5
NEUROCARE	4
CARDIAC CARE	3
DIAGNOSTIC IMAGING	2
ADMINISTRATIVE OFFICES	1
RADIATION ONCOLOGY/SUPPORT SERVICES DEPOT	G
MECHANICAL	B

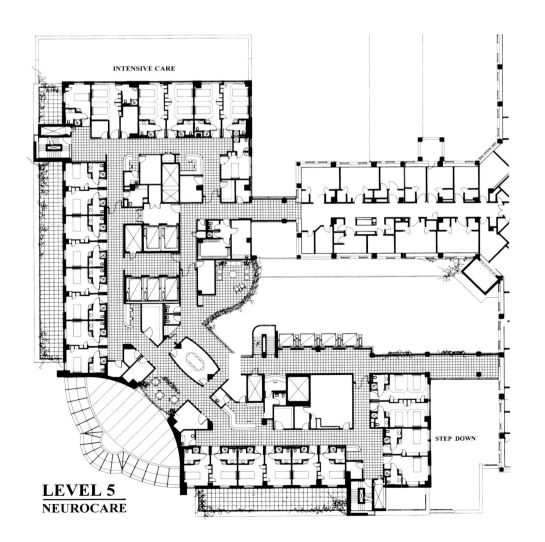

INTENSIVE CARE

STEP DOWN

LEVEL 5
NEUROCARE

Owner
University of Maryland Medical System

Data

Type of Facility
Hospital/inpatient care

Context
Hospital-based: 192 beds

Type of Construction
New

Area of Building
294,000 GSF

Cost of Construction
$70,000,000

Cost of Medical Equipment
$20,000,000

Status of Project
Completed October 1994

Credits

Architect
Zeidler Roberts Partnership, Inc., Architects
1025 St. Paul Street
Baltimore, Maryland

Structural Engineer
Oodesh Engineering, Inc.
Baltimore, Maryland

Mechanical/Electrical Engineer
Henry Adams, Inc.
Towson, Maryland

Landscape Architect
KCI Technologies
Hunt Valley, Maryland

Interior Design
Design Innerphase, Inc.
Silver Spring, Maryland

Interior Design of Atrium
Zeidler Roberts Partnership, Inc., Architects
Baltimore, Maryland

Vertical Transportation
Lerch Bates Hospital Group
Timonium, Maryland

Contractor
Turner Smoot Construction Company
Baltimore, Maryland

Photographer
Michael Dersin
Alexandria, Virginia

Kaiser Emeryville Medical Center

Oakland, California

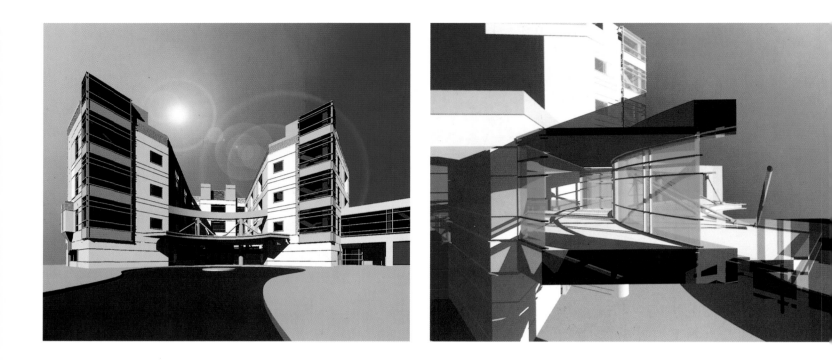

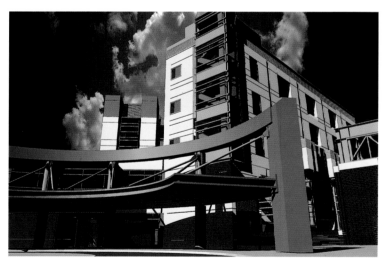

ARCHITECT'S STATEMENT

The one-million-square-foot flagship Kaiser Emeryville Medical Center responds to the rapidly changing health care environment by providing efficient adaptation to unknown future needs and symbolizing the partnership between community and provider. Modular organization of functions accommodates a variety of potential scenarios. An expandable footprint links diagnostic and "universal" nursing zones, each designed for variable acuity. Internal courtyards guide visitors, brighten rooms, and define "neighborhoods" within the hospital. Retail shops line a rejuvenated boulevard and revitalize an urban industrial neighborhood.

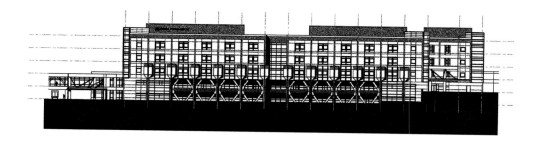

SOUTH ELEVATION

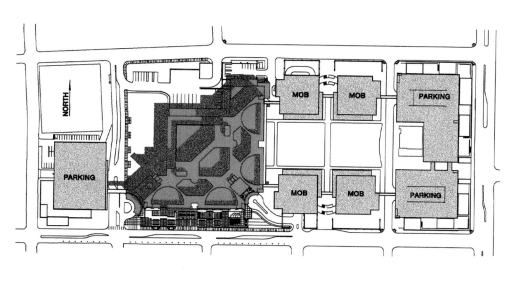

SITE PLAN

Owner

Kaiser Foundation Health Plan, Inc.

Data

Type of Facility

New hospital and multiuse medical campus

Context

Hospital-based: 191, 261, or 292 beds possible

Type of Construction

New

Area of Building

523,500 GSF (hospital and central utility plant only)

Cost of Construction

$130,000,000

Cost of Medical Equipment

$54,600,000 (including $1,600,000 furnishings)

Status of Project

Estimated completion date: January 1999

Credits

Architects

Joint Venture:
Stone Marraccini Patterson
One Market Place
Spear Street Tower, Fourth Floor
San Francisco, California 94105

DMJM Keating
3250 Wilshire Boulevard
Los Angeles, California 90010

Associate Architect

Michael Willis & Associates
246 First Street, Suite 200
San Francisco, California 94105

Structural Engineer

DMJM Keating
Los Angeles, California

Mechanical Engineer

Ted Jacob Engineering Group, Inc.
Oakland, California

Electrical Engineer

The Engineering Enterprise
Alameda, California

Civil Engineer

John T. Warren & Associates
Oakland, California

Landscape Architect

Chris Patillo Associates
Oakland, California

Interior Design

Simon Martin-Vegue
Winkelstein Moris
San Francisco, California

Cost Estimating

Adamson Associates
San Francisco, California

Parking Structure Consultant

International Parking Design, Inc.
Oakland, California

Lighting Consultant

Architectural Lighting Design
San Francisco, California

Acoustical Consultant

Charles M. Salter Associates, Inc.
San Francisco, California

Food Service Consultant

Cini-Little International
San Francisco, California

Elevators and Materials Management

Syska & Hennessey/Transport
Systems Group West
San Francisco, California

Security Consultant

Gibbs Associates
Fremont, California

Code and Fire Protection Consultant

Rolf Jensen & Associates, Inc.
Walnut Creek, California

Signage

Englund + Donnelly Design, Inc.
Walnut Creek, California

Contractor

Turner Construction
San Francisco, California

Photographer

Peter Xiques
San Francisco, California

LAC + USC Medical Center

Los Angeles, California

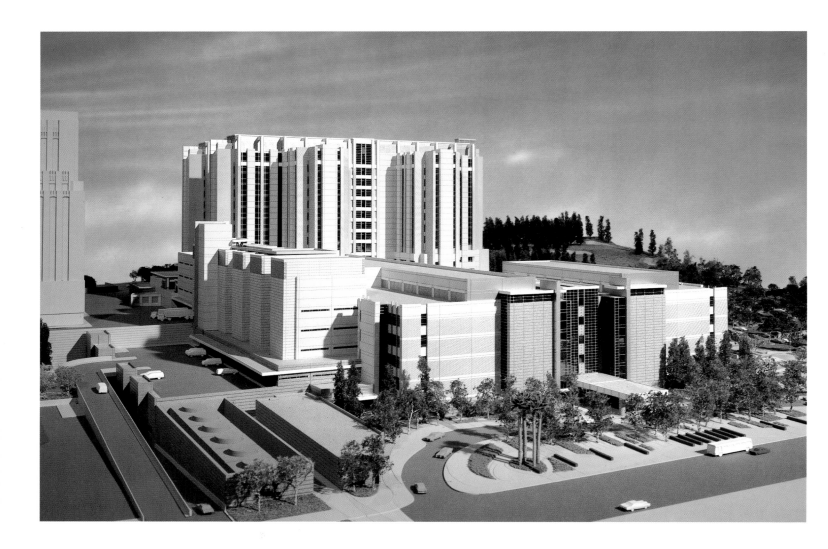

The new LAC + USC Medical Center, situated on an elevated site with the existing General Hospital, will become a symbol of institutional quality and civic pride, visible for miles in every direction. The replacement project will consolidate four existing acute-care hospitals and an outpatient building into one new state-of-the-art teaching hospital complex. This new complex includes a 15-story inpatient tower, a five-story outpatient clinic building, and a six-story diagnostic and treatment center, which will provide a "life boat" of emergency treatment facilities in the event of a major earthquake. This capability is made possible through an innovative base-isolation structural design that will allow this building to remain fully operational after a seismic event.

The medical center is positioned on its site to relate to the existing facility and to take advantage of the varied topography. Natural grade changes allow for distinct entries to the outpatient center to the south and to the inpatient tower to the north, which is on axis with the historic General Hospital.

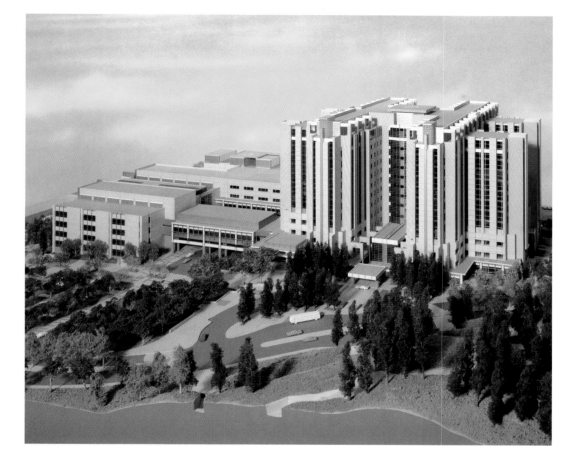

Owner

Los Angeles County Department of Health Services

Data

Type of Facility
Academic medical center

Context
Hospital-based: 946 beds

Type of Construction
New

Area of Building
2,135,559 GSF

Cost of Construction
Estimated: $995,238,520

Cost of Medical Equipment
Estimated: $150,776,520

Status of Project
Estimated date of completion: 2002

Credits

Architects

Associated Architects:

Lee, Burkhart, Liu
2890 Colorado Avenue
Santa Monica, California 90404

Hellmuth, Obata, Kassabaum
1655 26th Street, Suite 200
Santa Monica, California 90404

Structural Engineer
KPFF
Santa Monica, California

Mechanical/Electrical Engineer
Hayakawa Associates
Los Angeles, California

Cost Estimating
Adamson Associates
Santa Monica, California

Civil Engineering
Transmetrics
Los Angeles, California

Landscape Architect
Rios Associates
Los Angeles, California

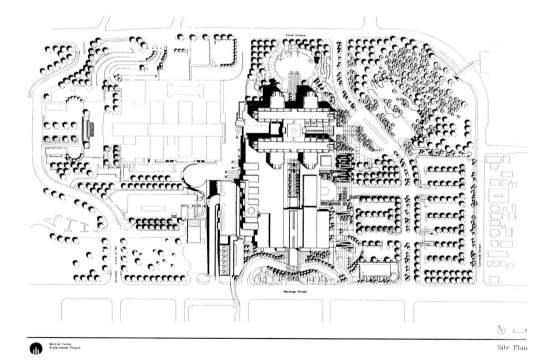

Medical Center
Replacement Project

Site Plan

Lahey Clinic North

Peabody, Massachusetts

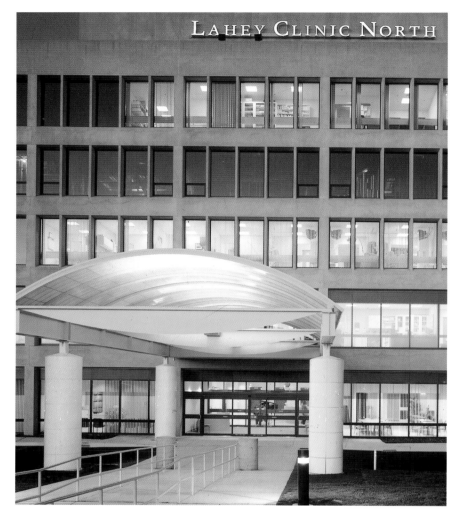

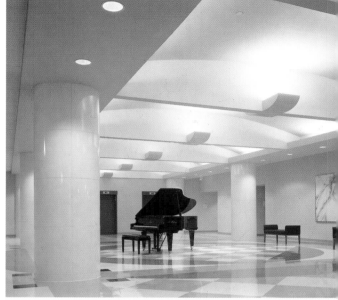

Lahey Clinic North is a ten-bed prototype hospital emphasizing ambulatory services, where providers from neighboring medical centers collaborate in providing the community with primary and specialty care, 24-hour emergency and inpatient services, and on-site diagnostic testing.

Using total quality management techniques and the charge to improve every aspect of the patient's encounter, the project team created innovative facilities, setting new standards for patient-focused care.

Distinctive design differentiates public spaces using vaulted ceilings, round columns, geometric floor patterns, and museum-quality artwork as way-finding features in this former bank building, extensively renovated to hospital standards.

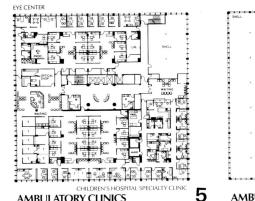

4 **AMBULATORY CLINICS**

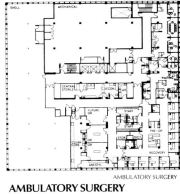

5 **AMBULATORY SURGERY**

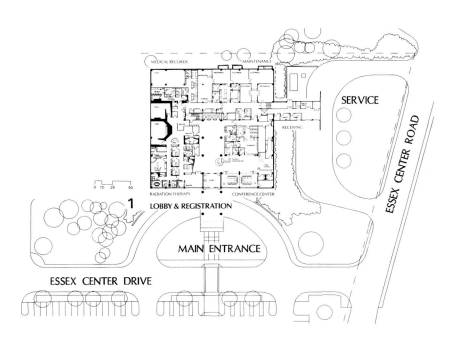

1 **LOBBY & REGISTRATION**

LakeWest Hospital

Willoughby, Ohio

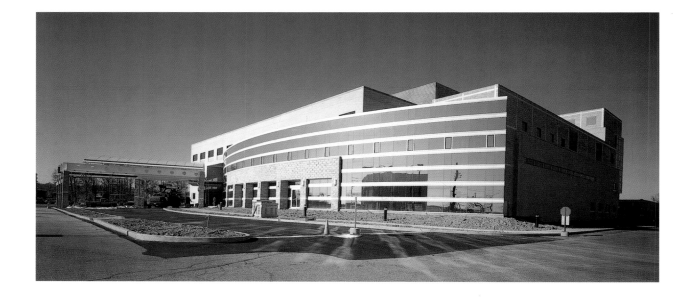

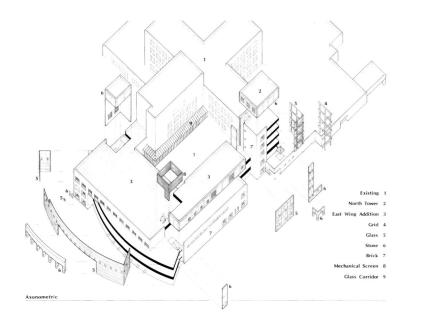

Existing 1
North Tower 2
East Wing Addition 3
Grid 4
Glass 5
Stone 6
Brick 7
Mechanical Screen 8
Glass Corridor 9

Axonometric

ARCHITECT'S STATEMENT

This hospital system constructed two major additions to the existing building, providing space to accommodate future needs. The North Tower addition is a four-level rectangular shape featuring reflective glass integrated with the existing building by use of matching brick and natural stone. The tower upgrades inpatient rooms and increases the ratio of private to semiprivate rooms.

The East Wing addition embraces the existing building and is punctuated by a new main entrance canopy. A two-level horizontal curved glass facade pierces the three-story brick volume. The East Wing houses the laboratory, cardiopulmonary, ambulatory surgery, community/meeting room, and a patient-focused medical/surgical unit.

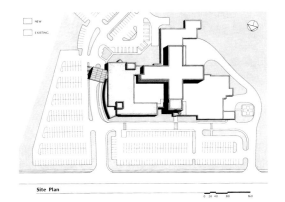

NEW
EXISTING

Site Plan

0 20 40 80 160

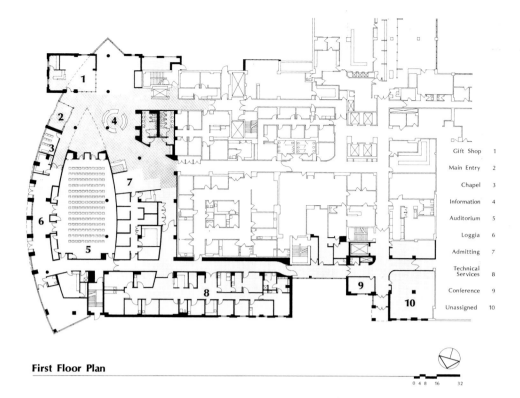

First Floor Plan

Gift Shop	1
Main Entry	2
Chapel	3
Information	4
Auditorium	5
Loggia	6
Admitting	7
Technical Services	8
Conference	9
Unassigned	10

0 4 8   16   32

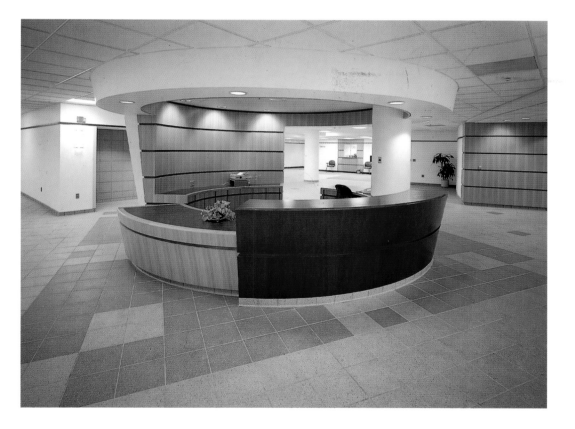

Owner

Lake Hospital System, Inc.

Data

Type of Facility

Acute care hospital

Context

Hospital-based: 191 beds

Type of Construction

New and renovation

Area of Building

115,284 GSF (86,180 new; 29,104 renovation)

Cost of Construction

Bid estimate: $12,559,007 ($10,592,886 new; $1,966,121 renovation)

Cost of Medical Equipment

Bid estimate: $613,370

Status of Project

Estimated completion date: August 1, 1995

Credits

Architect

Braun and Spice, Inc., Architects
7550 Lucerne Drive
Middleburg Heights, Ohio 44130

Structural Engineer

Barber & Hoffman, Inc.
Cleveland, Ohio

Mechanical/Electrical Engineer

Scheeser*Buckley*Mayfield, Inc.
Uniontown, Ohio

Civil Engineer

Lake, Inc.
Wickliffe, Ohio

Contractors

North Tower project:
John G. Johnson Construction
Chagrin Falls, Ohio

East Wing addition:
Panzica Construction Co.
Mayfield Village, Ohio

Photographers

North Tower project:
Alan Teufen
Medina, Ohio

East Wing addition:
Robert Heine
Cleveland, Ohio

Memorial Hospital Addition

Seymour, Indiana

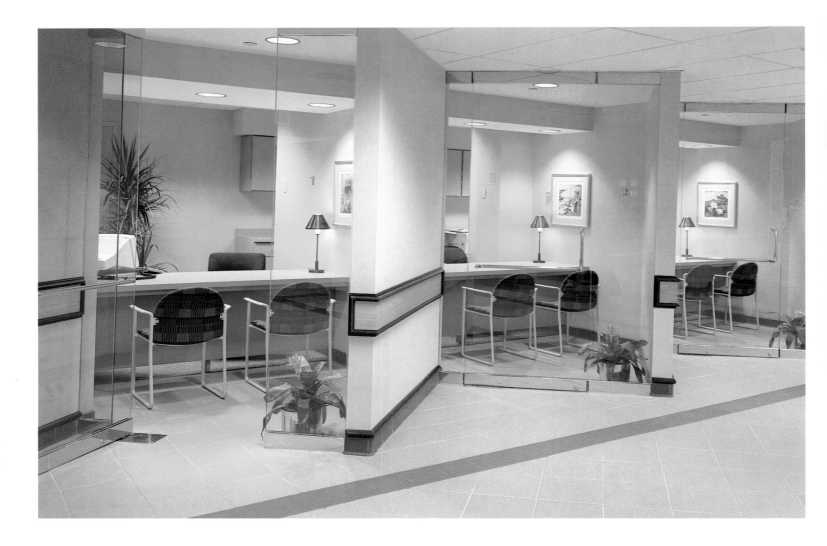

ARCHITECT'S STATEMENT

The primary goal of this project was to replace outdated, inaccessible diagnostic and treatment services and to redesign those services to position them for the shrinking inpatient market and the expanding outpatient market. Emergency, surgery, radiology, laboratory, and therapy services form the core of the newly designed environment.

Driven by a master plan, the scope of work included the site and utility expansion, a physician's office building, and renovation of the existing hospital for the compression of inpatient units and the expansion of various support services. Areas serving patients are organized along a linear internal "street" from the existing hospital through the diagnostic core and into the office building.

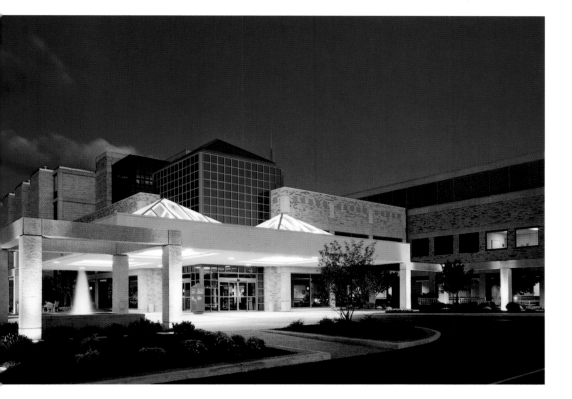

O w n e r
　Memorial Hospital

D a t a
　Type of Facility
　　Rural hospital addition

　Context
　　Hospital: 165 beds

　Type of Construction
　　New and renovation

　Area of Building
　　90,000 GSF (70,000 new; 20,000
　　renovation)

　Cost of Construction
　　$10,177,000
　　($9,027,000 new; $1,150,000
　　renovation)

　Cost of Medical Equipment
　　$5,581,000

　Status of Project
　　Completed October 1993

C r e d i t s
　Architect
　　BSA Design
　　6810 North Shadeland Avenue
　　Indianapolis, Indiana 46220

　*Structural/Mechanical/Electrical
　Engineer*
　　BSA Design
　　Indianapolis, Indiana

　Contractor
　　Jungclaus-Campbell
　　Indianapolis, Indiana

　Photographer
　　Mardan Photography
　　Indianapolis, Indiana

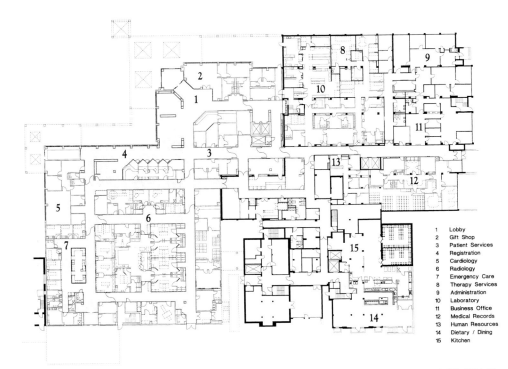

1　Lobby
2　Gift Shop
3　Patient Services
4　Registration
5　Cardiology
6　Radiology
7　Emergency Care
8　Therapy Services
9　Administration
10　Laboratory
11　Business Office
12　Medical Records
13　Human Resources
14　Dietary / Dining
15　Kitchen

FIRST FLOOR PLAN

MetroHealth Medical Center

Cleveland, Ohio

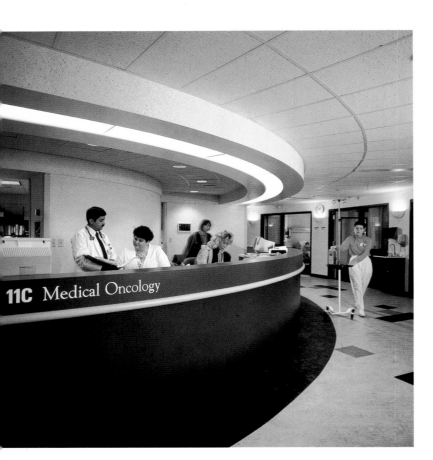

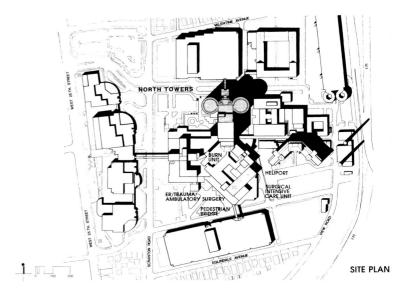

SITE PLAN

ARCHITECT'S STATEMENT

This project involves upgrading and modernizing 19 inpatient units in the east and west wings (the Towers) of the medical center's north building, plus constructing an addition for two new elevators, expanding patient/visitor lounges, and adding new con-ference/consultation facilities. The remodeled nursing units include: medical/surgical, oncology, pediatrics, mental health, obstetrics and gyne-cology, step-down, and a ten-bed critical care unit. The project includes expansion and renovation to provide for a 35-bed neonatal intensive care unit, a 43-bed obstetrical unit and newborn nurseries, and a 16-bed continuing care nursery.

The Towers' heating, ventilating, and air condi-tioning units were replaced, plus a new variable air volume system was added to all of the nursing units. The total mechanical replacement cost of $6 million had a payback of five years in energy savings. New electrical switch gear was added, along with new emergency power and a new fire alarm system. The 25-year-old building was updated in all mechanical and electrical areas.

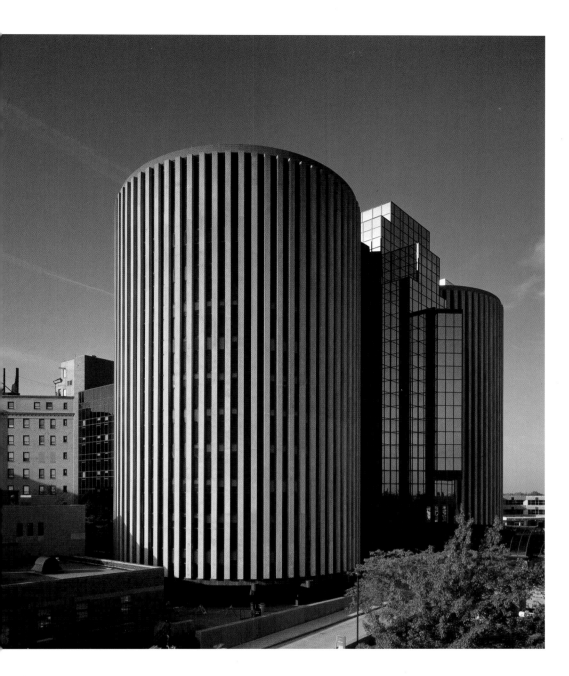

Owner
The MetroHealth System

Data

Type of Facility
Hospital

Context
Hospital-based: 511 beds

Type of Construction
Renovation and new

Area of Building
237,759 GSF (20,914 new;
216,845 renovation)

Cost of Construction
$22,000,000
($2,500,000 new; $19,500,000
renovation)

Cost of Medical Equipment
$4,000,000

Status of Project
Completed June 1995

Credits

Architect
HFP/Ambuske Architects
21403 Chagrin Boulevard
Cleveland, Ohio 44122

Structural Engineer
Barber & Hoffman, Inc.
Cleveland, Ohio

Mechanical/Electrical Engineer
Bacik Karpinski Associates, Inc.
Cleveland, Ohio

Interior Design
The Arris Group, Inc.
Cleveland, Ohio

Contractor
Dunlop & Johnston, Inc.
Cleveland, Ohio

Photographer
Roger Mastroianni
Cleveland, Ohio

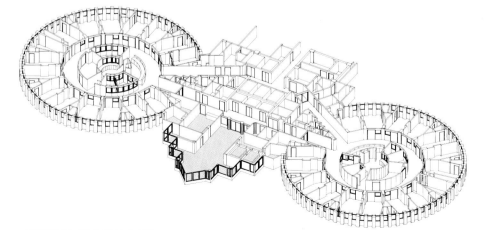

TYPICAL FLOOR PLAN

Newton Medical Center

Newton, Kansas

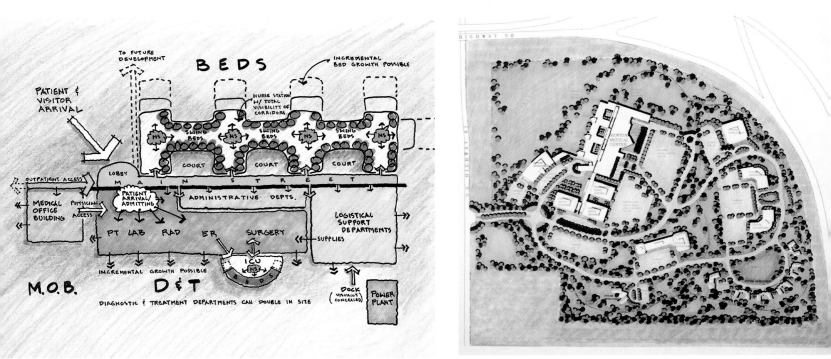

The key client objectives for the design of the replacement hospital were an emphasis on outpatient customer service, integration of physician practices, staffing efficiency, expansion capability, flexibility, and a strong visual presence. For easy patient access from both the contiguous clinics and other referrals from off site, the diagnostic and treatment departments are clustered near the main entrance, lobby, and admitting. Main Street, as an organizing device, becomes an armature around which all major hospital components are accessed. Wayfinding is easily evident and pleasant. Each major department has exterior wall frontage, allowing for individual expansion in small increments.

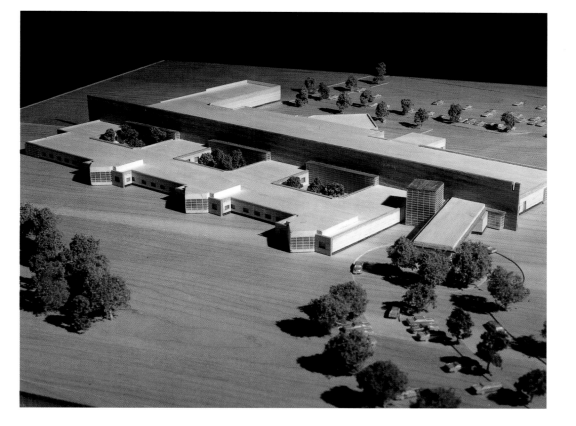

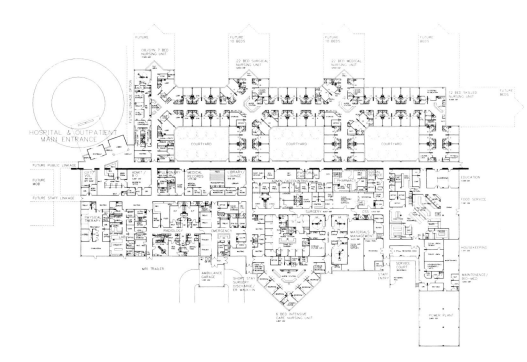

Owner
Newton Medical Center

Data

Type of Facility
Replacement community hospital

Context
Hospital-based: 66 beds

Type of Construction
New

Area of Building
114,168 GSF

Cost of Construction
$14,700,000

Cost of Medical Equipment
$1,400,000

Status of Project
Estimated completion date:
June 1996

Credits

Architect
Ellerbe Becket, Inc.
800 LaSalle Avenue
Minneapolis, Minnesota 55402-
2014

*Structural/Mechanical/Electrical
Engineer*
Ellerbe Becket, Inc.
Minneapolis, Minnesota

Food Service
Robert Rippe & Associates, Inc.
Minneapolis, Minnesota

Space Programming
Frank Zilm & Associates, Inc.
Kansas City, Missouri

Contractor
Ellerbe Becket Construction
Services
Minneapolis, Minnesota

Northwestern Memorial Hospital Redevelopment Project

Chicago, Illinois

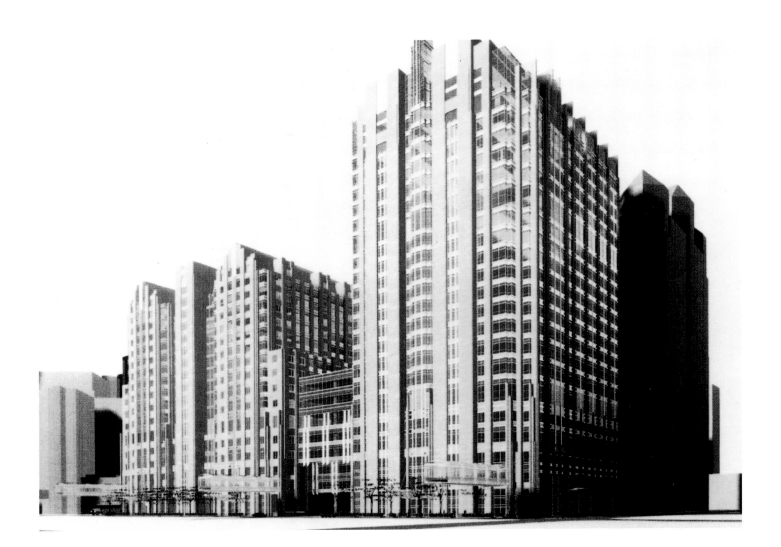

ARCHITECT'S STATEMENT

The new high-rise academic replacement hospital/ambulatory care center integrates a full range of inpatient and outpatient services into a single building concept on an urban site. Diagnostic and therapeutic services form a base for the double tower, with inpatient beds on one side and physician offices and faculty foundation on the other. The greatest challenge was to provide maximum patient care, convenience, and staff efficiency, while allowing for internal flexibility and seamless integration of inpatient and outpatient services. The facility complements the existing campus and expresses a sense of renewal while reinforcing the commitment to putting patients first.

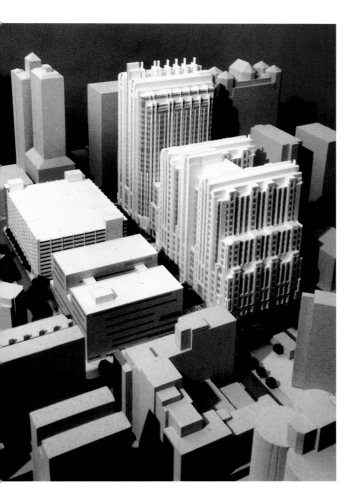

Owner
Northwestern Memorial Hospital

Data

Type of Facility
Replacement hospital/ambulatory
care

Context
Hospital-based: 496 beds

Type of Construction
New

Area of Building
2,100,000 GSF

Cost of Construction
Estimated: $380,000,000

Cost of Medical Equipment
Estimated: $100,000,000

Status of Project
Estimated completion date:
January 1999

Credits

Architect
Ellerbe Becket/Hellmuth, Obata
& Kassabaum, Inc. (HOK)
259 East Erie, Third floor
Chicago, Illinois 60611

Associate Architects
VOA Associates Incorporated
224 South Michigan Avenue,
Suite 1400
Chicago, Illinois 60604-2595

Johnson and Lee, LTD
828 South Wabash, Suite 210
Chicago, Illinois 60605

Structural Engineer
Hellmuth, Obata & Kassabaum
St. Louis, Missouri

Mechanical/Electrical Engineer
Environmental Systems Design
Chicago, Illinois

Civil Engineer
Globetrotters Engineering Corp.
Chicago, Illinois

Food Service
Robert Rippe & Associates, Inc.
Minneapolis, Minnesota

Vertical Transportation
Levee & Associates, Inc.
Bowie, Maryland

Lighting Consultant
Horton-Lees Lighting Design, Inc.
New York, New York

Contractor
Power/CRSS
Chicago, Illinois

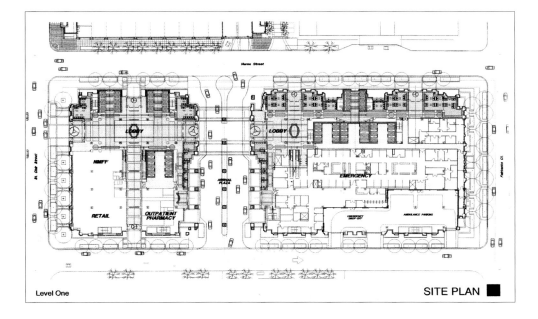

Level One

SITE PLAN ■

Planetree Demonstration Unit
Trinity Medical Center

Moline, Illinois

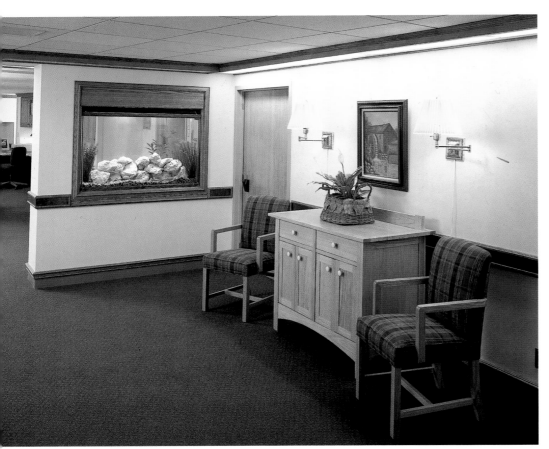

ARCHITECT'S STATEMENT

The project is a creative and inexpensive renovation of a nursing unit to demonstrate the Planetree model of care, which is intended to be incorporated into the replacement facility. The Planetree Model Unit serves as a "laboratory" and training ground for this new approach to the delivery of patient care. The ultimate goal is to identify the ideal healing environment and a patient-centered care program that empowers both the patient and staff.

A special effort was made to design a homelike environment that reflects Midwestern values and traditions. Areas such as the library and family room are particularly welcome additions to a traditional nursing unit. Light neutral finishes serve as a backdrop to colored upholstery used on the Shaker-style furniture. In order to transmit the message that individual attention has been crafted into the healing environment, the team custom-designed all furnishings, draperies, and the wall-covering borders.

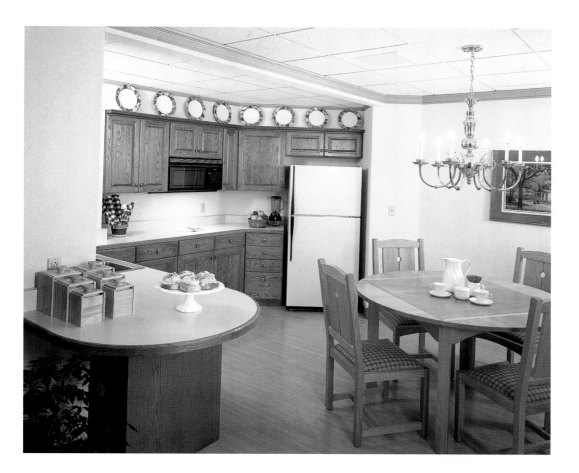

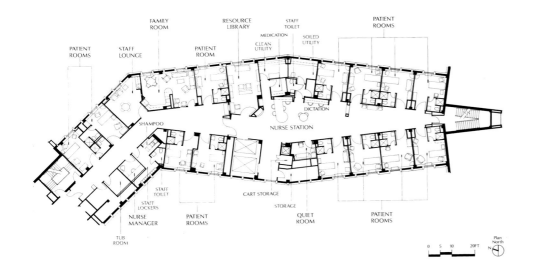

O w n e r
Trinity Regional Health System

D a t a

Type of Facility
Hospital

Context
Hospital-based: 13 beds

Type of Construction
Renovation

Area of Building
8,400 GSF

Cost of Construction
$400,000

Cost of Medical Equipment
$88,099 (furnishings—no medical equipment required)

Status of Project
Completed May 1993

C r e d i t s

Architect
Watkins Carter Hamilton Architects, Inc.
6575 West Loop South, Suite 300
Bellaire, Texas 77401

Mechanical/Electrical Engineer
Beling & Associates
Moline, Illinois

Planetree Consultant
Marc Schweitzer
San Francisco, California

Health Care Consultant
Dennis R. Moser & Associates
Kingwood, Texas

Contractor
C. E. Peterson & Sons, Inc.
Moline, Illinois

Photographer
Jud Haggard
Bellaire, Texas

Roanoke Memorial Hospital South Pavilion

Roanoke, Virginia

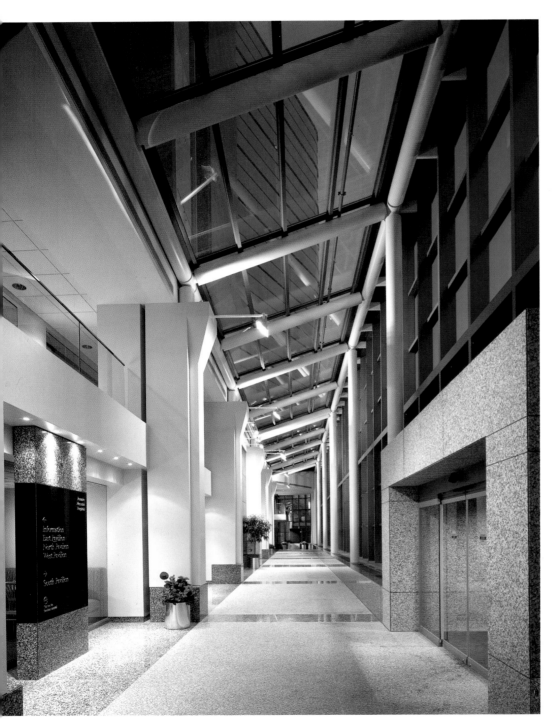

ARCHITECT'S STATEMENT

The project designers integrated the hospital's mission of delivering innovative, patient-focused care into a functional and contemporary design. Incorporating soothing and pleasant physical surroundings using space, light, color, and natural scenery, the design offers maximum comfort and reassurance for the patients, their families, and hospital staff. The nine-story wing, which can accommodate future expansion of five additional floors, was designed and built with a goal of cost containment. Through an extensive value-engineering process, all materials and equipment were selected for efficiency and durability. Likewise, floor plans were designed to make maximum use of space, minimizing costs to health care consumers.

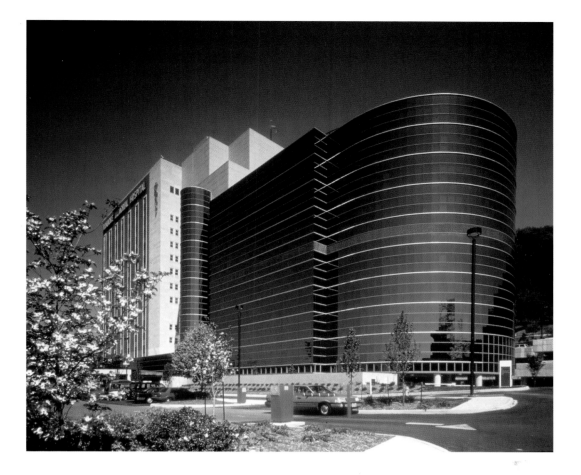

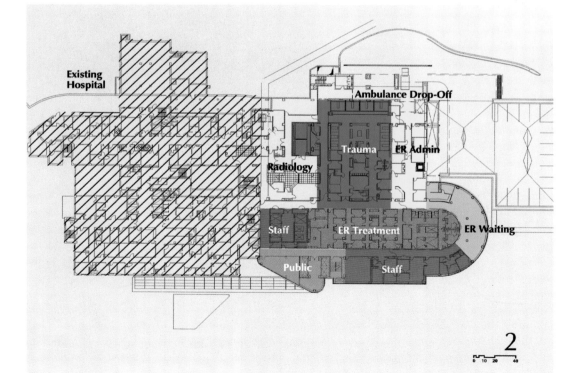

O w n e r

Carilion Health System
Roanoke, Virginia

D a t a

Type of Facility

Hospital addition

Context

Hospital-based: 123 beds

Type of Construction

New

Area of Building

335,000 GSF

Cost of Construction

$43,563,497

Cost of Medical Equipment

$19,000,000

Status of Project

Completed January 1994

C r e d i t s

Architect

JMGR Inc.
80 Monroe Avenue, Suite 900
Memphis, Tennessee 38103

Structural Engineer

JMGR Inc.
Memphis, Tennessee

Mechanical/Electrical Engineer

Newcomb & Boyd
Atlanta, Georgia

Civil Engineer

Mattern & Craig
Roanoke, Virginia

Interior Design

JMGR Inc.
Memphis, Tennessee

Facility Planner

Metis Associates, Ltd.
Chicago, Illinois

Medical Equipment Planner

JMGR Inc.
Memphis, Tennessee

Program Manager

The Adams Group
Rome, Georgia

Contractor

Beers Construction Company
Atlanta, Georgia

Photographer

Jeffrey Jacobs
Memphis, Tennessee

Roseville Hospital

Roseville, California

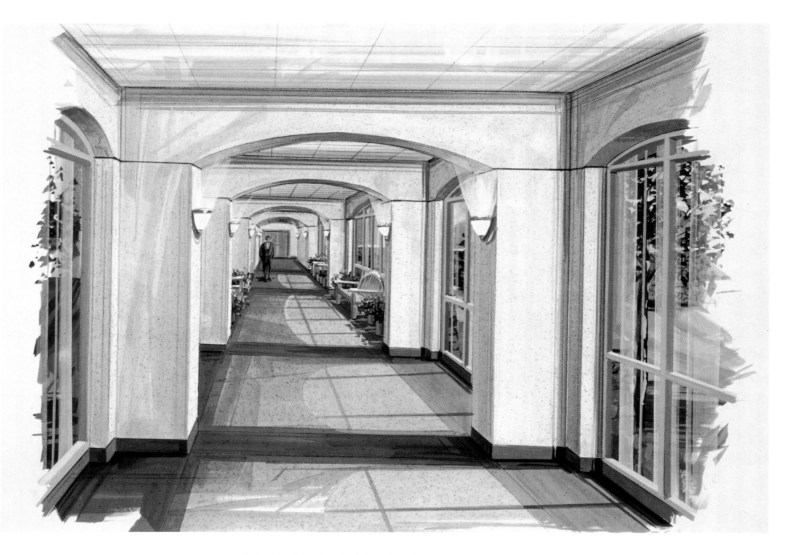

Several design challenges were faced in this project. The first was to promote healing through environmental design and thoughtful integration with the amenities of a carefully chosen site. The project team also sought to foster patient-centered care and to focus on the needs of patient and family in all aspects of their encounter with the facility. Ambulatory services had to be organized for convenient, direct access from one central arrival and registration point, and separate inpatient and outpatient work zones were required within centralized, integrated ancillary departments.

The design solution provides the convenience and accessibility demanded by ambulatory patients while recognizing the continual importance of delivering ambulatory and acute care efficiently in a cen-

tralized setting. The facility integrates inpatient and outpatient service under one roof, to maximize operational efficiency given projected patient volumes, and to deliver ambulatory care with the convenience traditionally associated with freestanding facilities.

This facility reflects the future of health care as the number of beds diminishes in favor of outpatient care. The future is also reflected in the integration of outpatient and inpatient services to achieve economies of operation. The uniqueness of the facility lies in its separation of the inpatient from ambulatory traffic in the workflow, and in the facility's inherent flexibility to accommodate change.

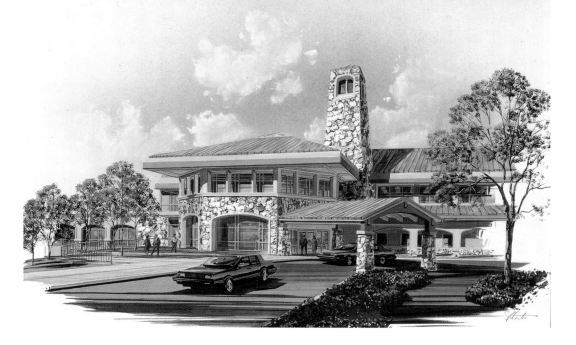

Owner
　　Roseville Hospital (Sutter Health
　　Affiliate)

Data
　Type of Facility
　　Medical Center

　Context
　　Hospital-based: 177 beds

Type of Construction
　New

Area of Building
　323,250 GSF

Cost of Construction
　$49,600,000

Cost of Medical Equipment
　$19,800,000

Status of Project
　Estimated completion date:
　December 1996

Credits
Architect
　HKS Architects, Inc.
　3420 Ocean Park Boulevard,
　Suite 3080
　Santa Monica, California 90405

Associate Architect
　Williams Paddon Architects
　& Planners, Inc.
　2240 Douglas Boulevard,
　Suite 250
　Roseville, California 95661

Structural Engineer
　Cole/Yee/Schubert & Associates
　Sacramento, California

Mechanical/Electrical Engineer
　Smith Seckman Reid, Inc.
　Nashville, Tennessee

Civil Engineer
　Omni-Means
　Roseville, California

Interior Designer
　Kelly Design Group
　Roseville, California

Medical Equipment Consultant
　Facilities Development, Inc.
　Phoenix, Arizona

Contractor
　McCarthy=HMH
　Sacramento, California

Photographer
　Rick Grunbaum
　(model photography)
　Dallas, Texas

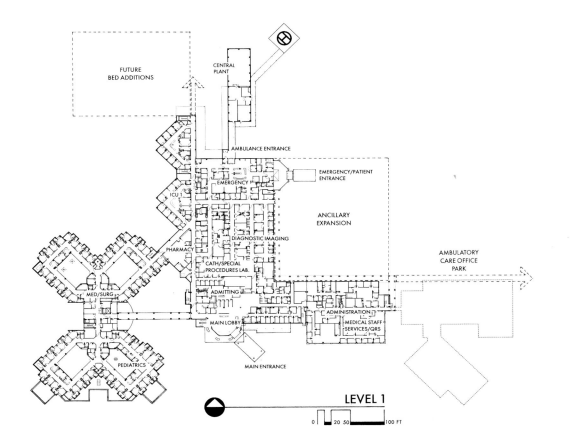

LEVEL 1

0　20 50　　100 FT

Rush-Copley Medical Center

Aurora, Illinois

Owner

Copley Memorial Hospital

Data

Type of Facility

New campus and medical center of regional system

Context

Hospital-based: 144 beds

Type of Construction

New

Area of Building

261,700 GSF
(plus 85,900-GSF medical office building)

Cost of Construction

$60,600,000

Cost of Medical Equipment

$2,200,000

Status of Project

Estimated date of completion: November 1995

Credits

Architect

O'Donnell Wicklund Pigozzi and Peterson Architects, Inc. (OWP&P)
570 Lake Cook Road
Deerfield, Illinois 60015

Structural Engineer

OWP&P
Deerfield, Illinois

Mechanical Engineer

Environmental Systems Design, Inc.
Chicago, Illinois

Electrical Engineer

Dickerson Engineering, Inc.
Niles, Illinois

Landscape Architect

Don Halam Associates
Chicago, Illinois

Civil Engineer

Rempe-Sharpe & Associates, Inc.
Geneva, Illinois

Cost Estimating

Construction Cost Systems, Inc.
Lombard, Illinois

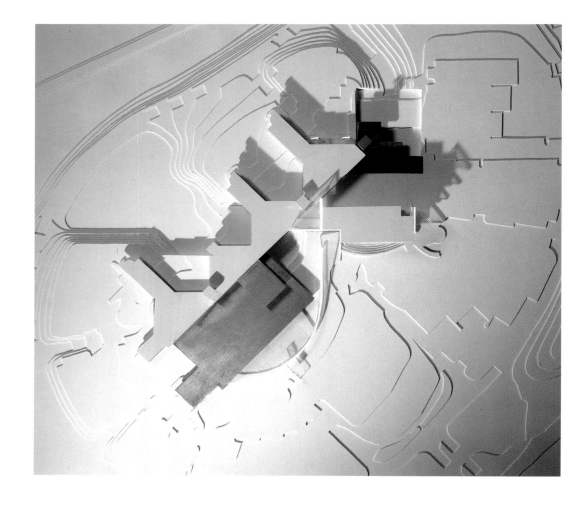

ARCHITECT'S STATEMENT

This new facility is designed to bring the components of care to the patient. The concept breaks the traditional hospital into four major parts. This plan allows for independent identity and access for each component. The technical center (diagnostic and therapy services) has an entrance allowing each patient to park, check in, get access to care, and exit in less than a 175-foot travel distance. The hospitality accommodations are located along the clinical-circulation spine, oriented to the pastoral side of the site, which provides the patients with a comforting view of a natural setting. The medical office building and corporate office house administrative services and private offices for physicians. The service component is strategically positioned for discretion and future expansion.

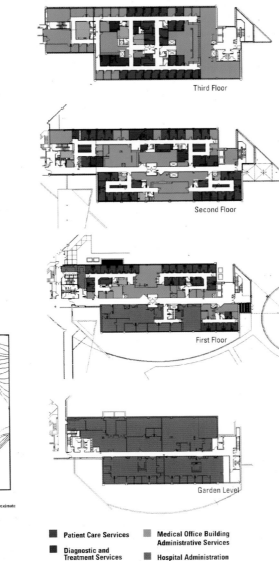

Third Floor

Second Floor

First Floor

Garden Level

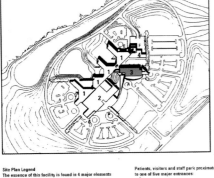

Site Plan Legend
The essence of this facility is found in 4 major elements

1 **Hospitality Accommodations**
for the nursing care of overnight patients

2 **Technical Center**
for the diagnosis and treatment of all patients

3 **Corporate & Medical Office Building**
for administration and physicians' suites

4 **Services**
support departments, service docks and power plant

Patients, visitors and staff park proximate to one of five major entrances:

A Public Entrance
B Patient Entrance
C Emergency Entrance
D Oncology Center
E Rehabilitation Center

Other site features or entrances:

F Service Docks
G Medical Office Building Entrance

■ **Patient Care Services**

■ **Diagnostic and Treatment Services**

■ **Support and Services**

■ **Medical Office Building Administrative Services**

■ **Hospital Administration and Services**

Credits (continued)

Owner's Representative and Equipment Consultant

American Medical Design
Corporation
Chicago, Illinois

Hospital Contractor

Mortenson/Schwendener
Joint Venture
Aurora, Illinois

Medical Office Building Contractor

Pepper Construction Company
Chicago, Illinois

St. Joseph Medical Center, Admitting Department

Tacoma, Washington

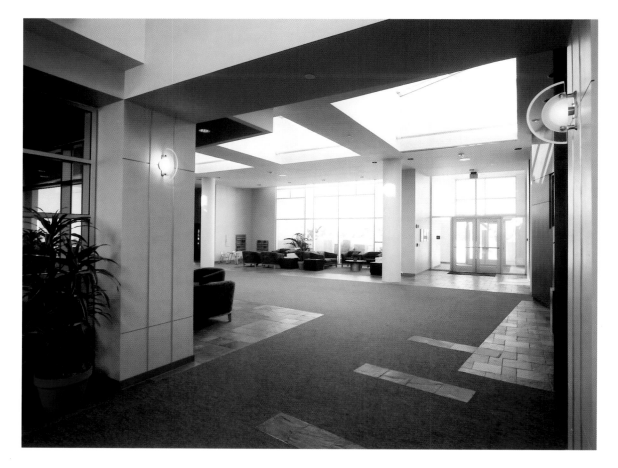

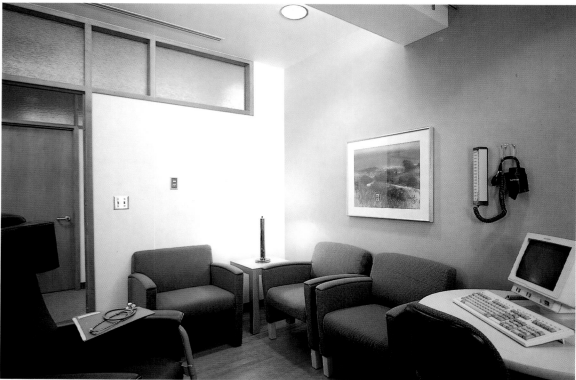

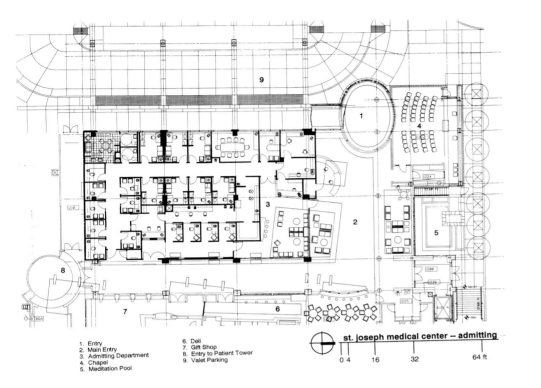

1. Entry
2. Main Entry
3. Admitting Department
4. Chapel
5. Meditation Pool
6. Deli
7. Gift Shop
8. Entry to Patient Tower
9. Valet Parking

st. joseph medical center -- admitting

0 4   16   32   64 ft

O w n e r
Franciscan Health System

D a t a
Type of Facility
Hospital

Context
Hospital-based

Type of Construction
New

Area of Project
5,421 GSF

Cost of Construction
$777,977

Cost of Medical Equipment
$150,000

Status of Project
Completed September 1993

C r e d i t s
Architect
Buffalo Design, Inc.
1501 Western Avenue, Suite 500
Seattle, Washington 98101

Architect of Record
Heery International
999 Peachtree Street N.E.
Atlanta, Georgia 30367

Structural Engineer
Anderson Bjornstad Kane Jacobs, Inc.
Seattle, Washington

Mechanical/Electrical Engineer
Heery International
Atlanta, Georgia

Master Planning
David Chambers, HNTB
Seattle, Washington

Interior Designer
Buffalo Design, Inc.

Contractor
Sellen Construction
Seattle, Washington

Photographer
Chris Eden, Eden Arts
Seattle, Washington

ARCHITECT'S STATEMENT

Traditional hospital admitting departments are often the source of much confusion and aggravation for patients. In response to this, the architects and interior designers worked to centralize all admitting procedures, from administration to diagnostics. Pre-admitting activity is centered in private, nonclinical rooms. The staff comes to the patient for testing and record-taking, instead of the patient to the staff. Everything—from financial counseling to educational videos—is available in this nonthreatening environment.

A second group of express check-in rooms is conveniently located between the patient waiting and staff support spaces. On the morning of admission, patients may register here and pass through to acute care areas in a matter of minutes.

St. Luke's Medical Center Galleria and Outpatient Service Addition

Milwaukee, Wisconsin

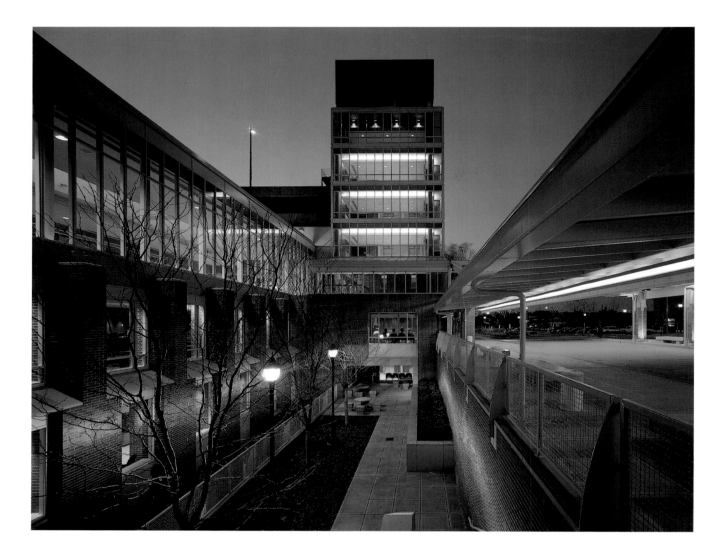

ARCHITECT'S STATEMENT

St. Luke's Medical Center has multiple existing entrances because of additions and renovations, giving the campus a circuitous circulation system and no apparent main entrance. A major challenge was to provide clinical services while integrating a simple and identifiable organizational system around existing departments.

The outpatient addition is inserted between existing facilities, echoing their simple shapes and horizontal form. Clad predominantly in brick with stone detailing, the addition's enclosure is composed of a series of opaque and transparent forms that reflect its context in form and materiality. Patients, visitors, and staff enter the facility through a skylit lobby adjacent to and overlooking a terraced courtyard. The court-

yard provides natural light to secondary public spaces on lower levels. Each of these lower lobbies recalls the primary entry space through the use of similar materials and orientation to common spaces and landmarks. This strategy brings the threshold of departments on lower floors up to the main entry.

The lobby leads directly into the galleria, a linear organizational element that provides a public circulation and waiting zone designed to serve outpatient services and later phases of inpatient development. Individual departments are identified by a crossing skylight above the sculpted ceilings which serve as light reflectors back into the galleria.

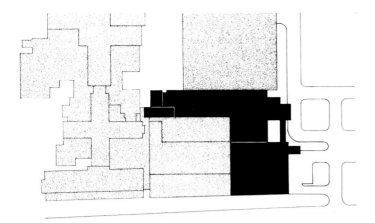

Figure/Ground

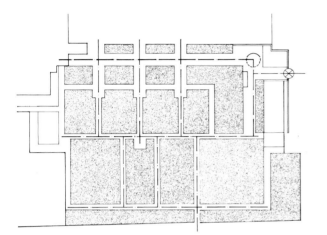

Circulation

O w n e r
St. Luke's Medical Center

D a t a
Type of Facility
Hospital outpatient facility

Context
Hospital-based: 711 beds

Type of Construction
New and renovation

Area of Building
208,000 GSF (171,000 new;
37,000 renovation)

Cost of Construction
38,000,000 ($32,900,000 new;
$5,100,000 renovation)

Cost of Medical Equipment
$3,800,000

Status of Project
Completed addition:
December 1992
Completed renovation:
December 1993

C r e d i t s
Architect
Bobrow/Thomas & Associates
(BTA)
1001 Westwood Boulevard
Los Angeles, California 90024

*Structural/Mechanical/Electrical
Engineer*
Schmidt, Garden & Erikson, Inc.
Chicago, Illinois

Landscape Architect
The Jacob Braun Company
Tulsa, Oklahoma

Interior Design
Public Spaces:
BTA
Los Angeles, California
Technical Spaces:
Davenish Associates, Inc.
Madison, Wisconsin

Medical Equipment Planning
Mitchell International
Skokie, Illinois

Construction Manager
Oscar J. Boldt Construction
Company
Appleton, Wisconsin

Photographers
Wayne E. Cable
Chicago, Illinois

Grant Mudford
Los Angeles, California

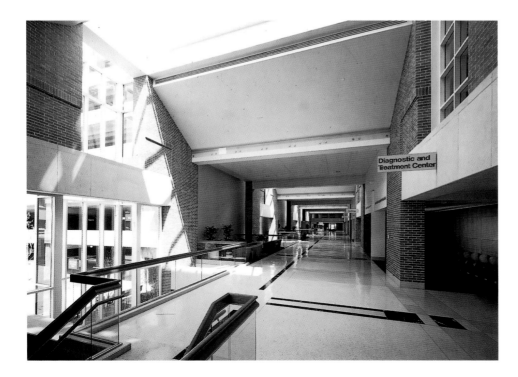

St. Vincent's Medical Center Services Building and Clinical Services Building

Jacksonville, Florida

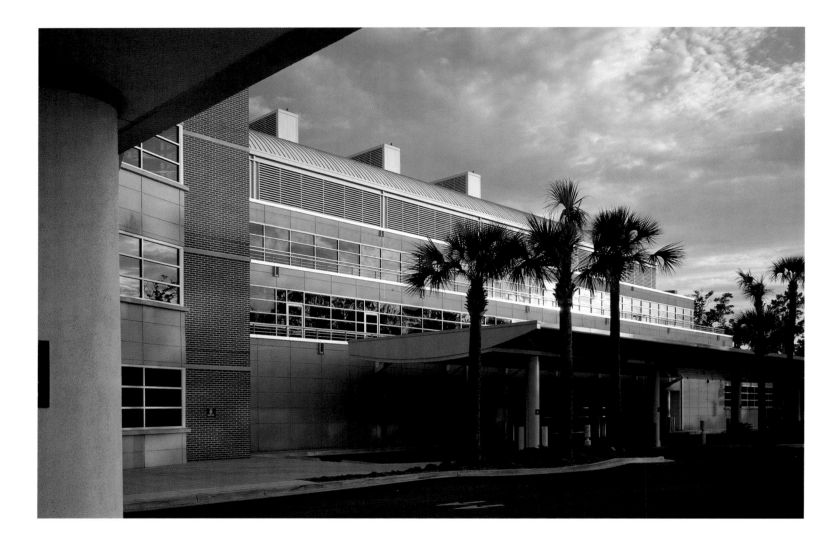

ARCHITECT'S STATEMENT

Replacement and expansion have, in effect, redeveloped this hospital on its existing campus. The site is essentially landlocked, located in a historic preservation district on the edge of the waterfront.

The new Services and Clinical Services buildings are designed to enhance flagship services and recapture vacated space for retrofit as an ambulatory care mall. The Services building consolidates the receiving, storage, dietary, laboratory, and ancillary departments along the nonpublic edge of the campus. The Clinical Services building houses an emergency department designed for 60,000 annual visits. Circulation modes are carefully segregated: pedestrian from vehicular, ambulatory from ambulance, emergency room parking from general parking. The remainder of the building provides for intensive care, LDRP, diagnostic cardiology, and future expansion.

The DePaul building, also part of the redevelopment, is a multi-use, joint-venture project featuring a nine-story tower spanning the public thoroughfare to the hospital's main entry, elevated two stories above. The lower three levels connect directly to the hospital, enabling the expansion of diagnostic and treatment services. The upper six stories function as a medical office building.

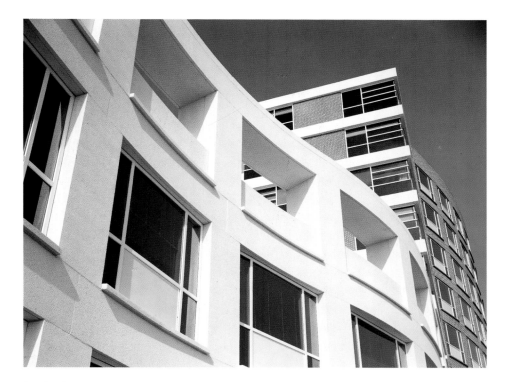

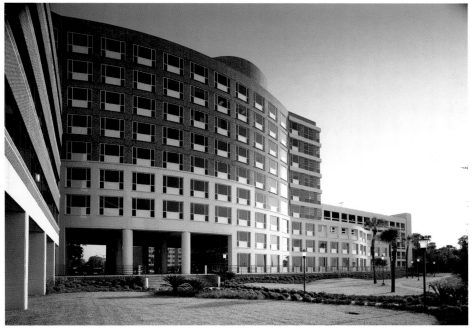

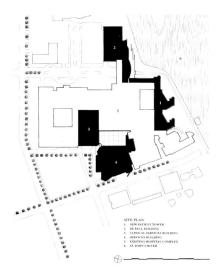

SITE PLAN
1. NEW PATIENT TOWER
2. DE PAUL BUILDING
3. CLINICAL SERVICES BUILDING
4. SERVICES BUILDING
5. EXISTING HOSPITAL COMPLEX
6. ST. JOHN'S RIVER

Owner
St. Vincent's Medical Center

Data

Type of Facility
Building addition to medical center, services, and clinical facility

Context
Hospital-based: 528 beds

Type of Construction
New

Area of Building
226,000 GSF

Cost of Construction
$31,400,000

Cost of Medical Equipment
Not available

Status of Project
Completed April 1992

Credits

Architect
CANNON
One Independent Drive
Jacksonville, Florida 32202

Structural Engineer
Siebold, Syndow & Elsanbaum
St. Louis, Missouri

Mechanical/Electrical Engineer
Smith Seckman Reid, Inc.
Ft. Lauderdale, Florida

Contractor
The Auchter Company, Inc.
Jacksonville, Florida

Photographer
Robert Pettus
St. Louis, Missouri

Silverton Hospital

Silverton, Oregon

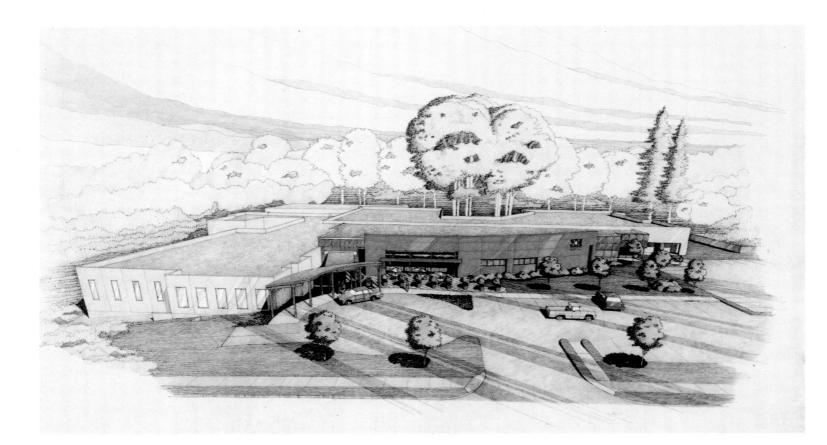

This addition to a small community hospital replaces all inpatient care, surgery, same-day unit, dietary, and miscellaneous support. The design is focused on patients and families. Orientation is achieved by using a double "spine" organization, which separates the public from staff. The entrance is through a welcoming courtyard containing an outdoor cafe, and the public spine is enlivened with daylight, lounges, color, galleries, and views of nature.

Inpatient areas are healing environments that focus on outdoor gardens through large wood-framed windows. All lighting is indirect. Natural wood is used for cabinets and railings, and soft colors are prevalent.

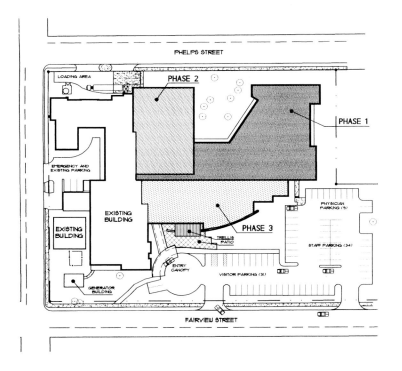

SITE PLAN

0 15 30 45 75   N

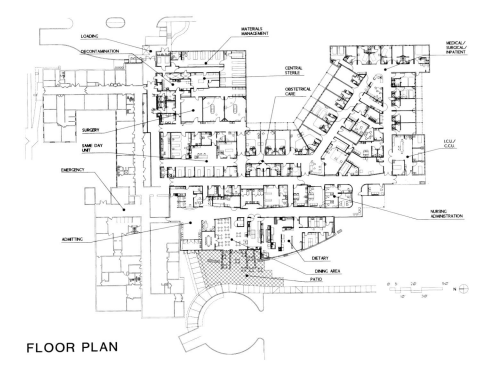

FLOOR PLAN

0 10 20 30 50   N

Owner
Silverton Hospital

Data

Type of Facility
Community hospital

Context
Hospital-based: 34 beds

Type of Construction
New and renovation

Area of Building
40,000 GSF (38,000 new; 2,000 renovation)

Cost of Construction
$4,879,000 ($4,579,000 new construction; $300,000 renovation)

Cost of Medical Equipment
$983,000

Status of Project
Estimated completion date: August 1995

Credits

Architect
Clark/Kjos Architects
133 SW Second Avenue, Suite 410
Portland, Oregon 97204

Structural Engineer
VLMK Associates
Portland, Oregon

Mechanical Engineer
Manfull-Curtis
Portland, Oregon

Electrical Engineer
Interface Engineering, Inc.
Portland, Oregon

Interior Design
Carla Fox, Interior Planning and Design
Portland, Oregon

Contractor
Andersen Construction Co., Inc.
Portland, Oregon

Sutter Davis Hospital

Davis, California

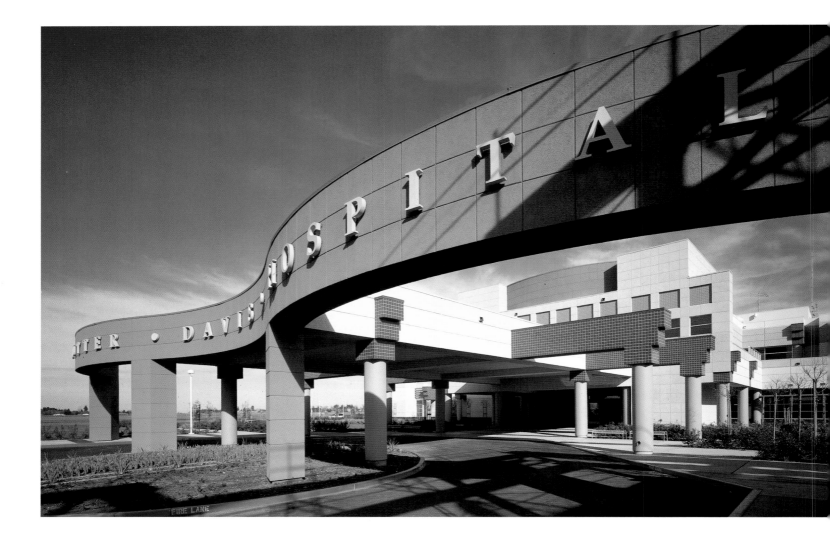

ARCHITECT'S STATEMENT

This two-story facility serves three small communities in northern California. Placing major emphasis on the outpatient, the owner's primary goal was to design an "outpatient facility with beds." Inpatient beds in six-bed, single-room care suites are located on the second floor. Outpatient areas are on the first floor for access and convenience. Inpatients on the first floor use a separate corridor from outpatients and visitors. Designed to appear high-tech, yet retain the small community feel, the facility is organized around a courtyard that creates a tranquil environment for quality health care.

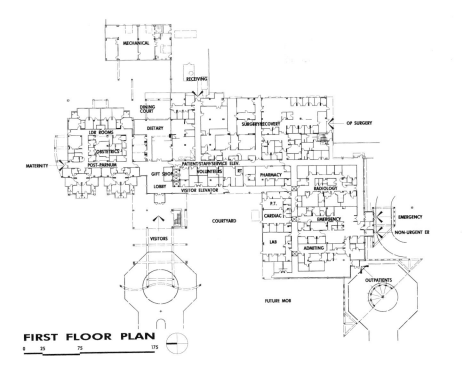

FIRST FLOOR PLAN

0   25   75   175

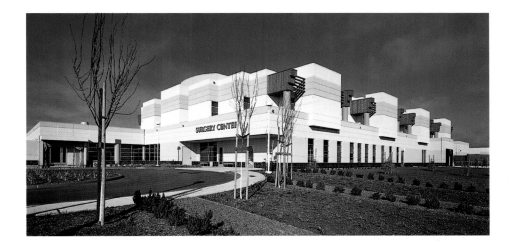

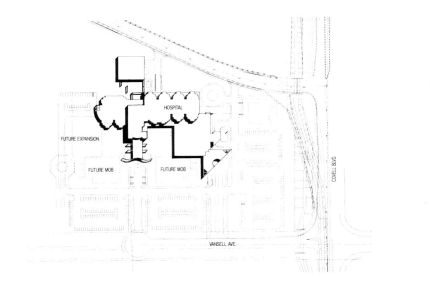

SITE PLAN

Owner

Sutter Health System

Data

Type of Facility

Outpatient-based community hospital

Context

Hospital-based: 54 beds

Type of Construction

New

Area of Building

95,490 GSF

Cost of Construction

$16,214,505 (does not include radiographic equipment)

Cost of Medical Equipment

Not available

Status of Project

Completed September 1994

Credits

Architect

Henningson, Durham & Richardson, Inc.
8404 Indian Hills Drive
Omaha, Nebraska 68114

Structural Engineer

Cole, Yee and Schubert
Sacramento, California

Mechanical/Electrical Engineer

Henningson, Durham & Richardson, Inc.
Omaha, Nebraska

Civil Engineer

Cunningham Engineering
Davis, California

Landplanners/Landscape Consultant

SWA Group
Sausalito, California

Dietary Planner

Tom Morrow
Lincoln, Nebraska

Contractor

John F. Otto, Inc.
Sacramento, California

Photographer

Ronald Moore Photography
Tustin, California

Yuma Regional Medical Center

Yuma, Arizona

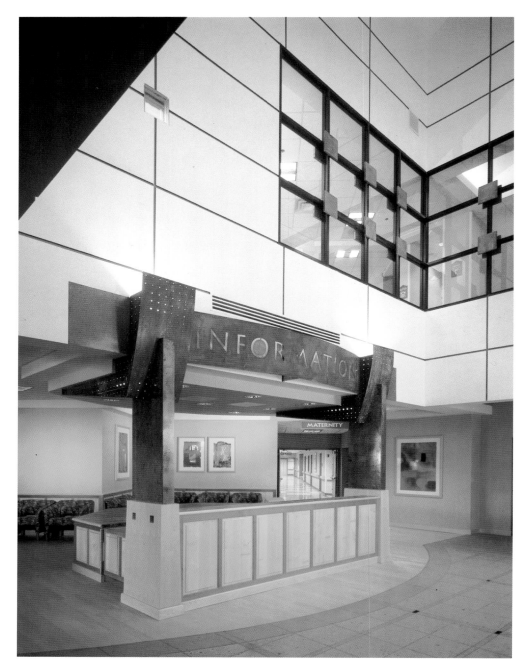

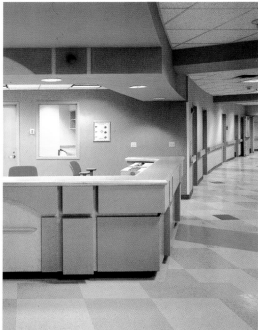

ARCHITECT'S STATEMENT

The addition and renovation provided expanded maternal and child care for this regional medical center. The objective was to design a building that would blend architecturally with the existing facility but still be perceived as independent from it. The design solution relates well to the existing campus, while allowing the introduction of new forms and materials, broadening the architectural language of the campus. A separate entry and lobby area contribute to the building's sense of independence.

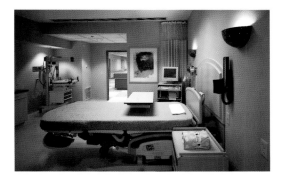

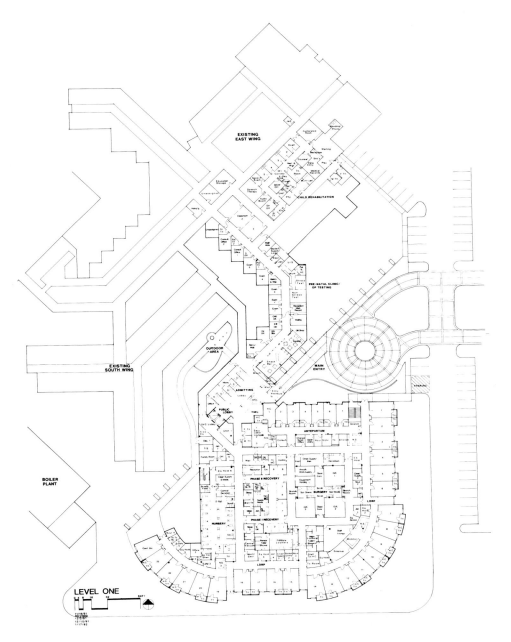

LEVEL ONE

O w n e r
Yuma Regional Medical Center

D a t a
Type of Facility
Hospital and outpatient clinics

Context
Hospital-based: 54 beds

Type of Construction
New and renovation

Area of Building
95,821 GSF (79,321 new;
16,500 renovation)

Cost of Construction
$9,852,592

Cost of Medical Equipment
$470,000

Status of Project
Completed April 1994

C r e d i t s
Architect
HKS, Inc.
700 N. Pearl, Suite 1100
Dallas, Texas 75201

Structural Engineer
HKS, Inc.
Dallas, Texas

Mechanical / Electrical Engineer
Smith Seckman Reid, Inc.
Nashville, Tennessee

Civil Engineer
Gookin Engineers
Scottsdale, Arizona

Interior Design
Squaw Peak Design Associates
Phoenix, Arizona

Construction Manager / Contractor
McCarthy
Phoenix, Arizona

Photographer
Wes Thompson
Keller, Texas

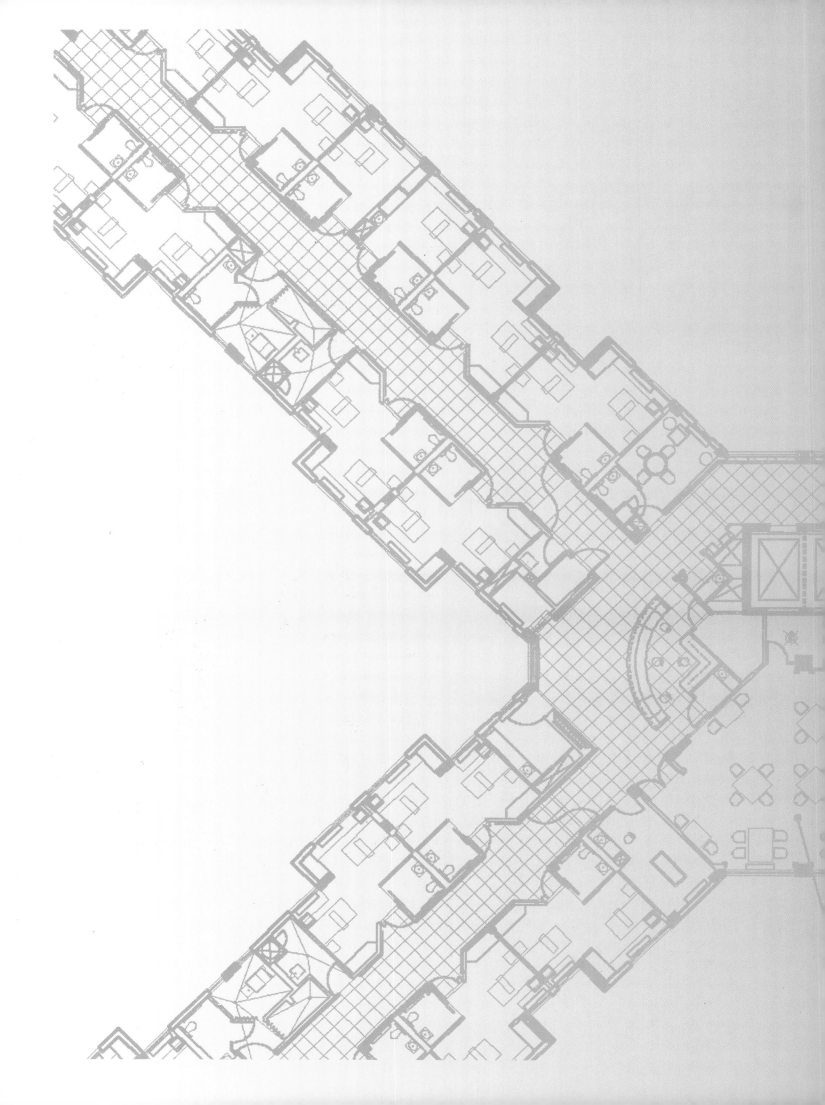

Long-Term Care Facilities

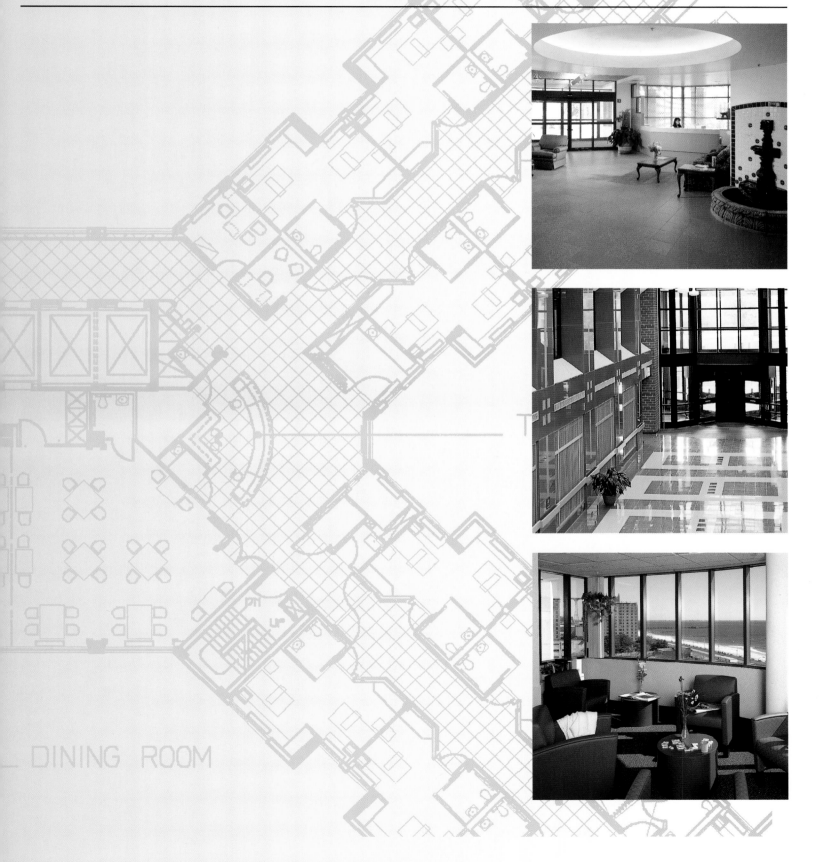

DINING ROOM

Harold & Patricia Toppel Center for Life Enhancement at Miami Jewish Home and Hospital for the Aged

Miami, Florida

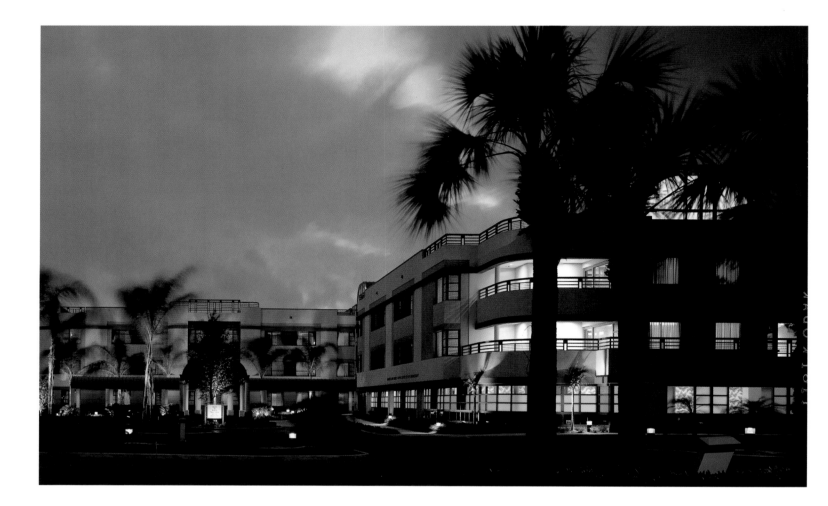

ARCHITECT'S STATEMENT

The Harold & Patricia Toppel Center for Life Enhancement is a 174-bed skilled-nursing replacement building. The three-story facility offers a flexibly sized nursing unit that can expand or contract as needed (from ten to 40 beds), with spatial organization to promote such versatility. Three unique room environments are available; two specialty ten-capacity wings with private parlor suites, unusually private semiprivate suites, and short-term-stay hospital rooms. The center links directly to an adjacent occupied 120-bed building forming an interconnected inner and outer quadrangle around new "relearning to walk" gardens. Stucco, tile, and decorative metal are intended to resemble the Miami Beach-style apartment houses, an exuberant and colorful character for a nursing home.

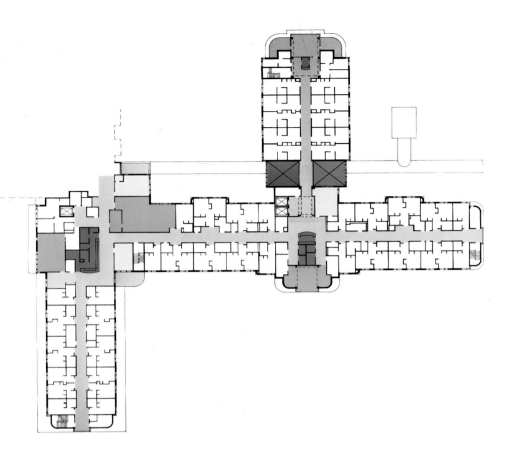

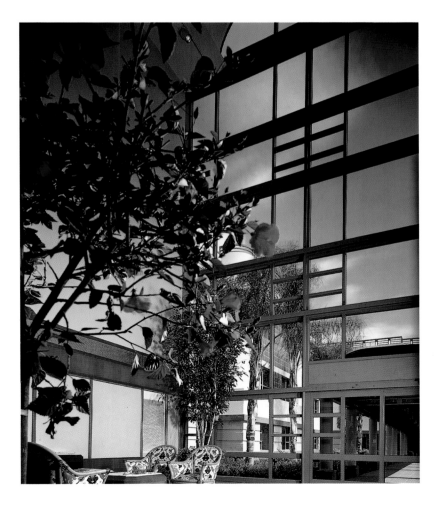

Owner

Miami Jewish Home and Hospital
for the Aged at Douglas Gardens

Data

Type of Facility

Long-term care, rehabilitation,
and skilled-nursing facility

Context

Freestanding

Type of Construction

New

Area of Building

113,000 GSF

Cost of Construction

$11,000,000

Cost of Medical Equipment

$370,000

Status of Project

Completed 1992

Credits

Architect

The Geddis Partnership, Architects,
Planners, Interior Designers
2023 Summer Street
Stamford, Connecticut 06905

Structural Engineer

Cantor/Seinuk/Puig
Miami, Florida

Mechanical Engineer

Juan Lagomasino, P.E.
Miami, Florida

Electrical Engineer

Nelson Vital, P.E.
Miami, Florida

Contractor

Turner Construction Company
Miami, Florida

Photographer

Dan Cornish
New Canaan, Connecticut

Shorefront Jewish Geriatric Center

Brooklyn, New York

Owner
Metropolitan Jewish Healthcare
System

Data
Type of Facility
Residential health care facility

Context
Freestanding

Type of Construction
New

Area of Building
175,000 GSF

Cost of Construction
$31,500,000

Cost of Medical Equipment
$2,300,000

Status of Project
Completed

Credits
Architect
Landow and Landow Architects,
P.C., AIA
3000 Marcus Avenue
Lake Success, New York 11042

Structural Engineer
The Office of Irwin G. Cantor
New York, New York

Mechanical/Electrical Engineer
Edwards and Zuck
New York, New York

Geotechnical Engineer
Mueser Rutledge
New York, New York

Hydraulics Engineer
Carmine E. Procassini, P.E.
New York, New York

Environmental Psychologist
Lorraine G. Hiatt
New York, New York

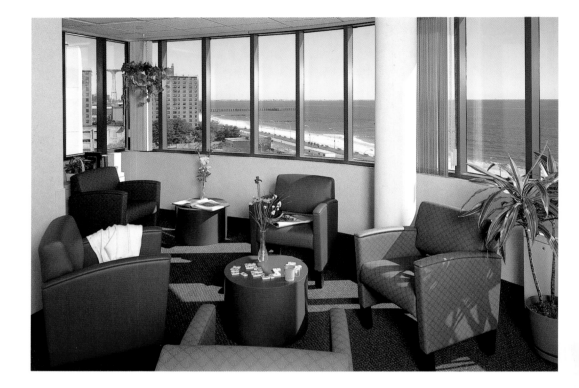

ARCHITECT'S STATEMENT

This 360-bed residential health care facility serves a population with medical and cognitive impairments including Alzheimer's disease and related disorders. The project is located on the boardwalk, overlooking the Atlantic Ocean, next to the converted hotel that housed the residents for almost half a century.

The challenge was to allow the original building to remain in operation during construction without sacrificing function or aesthetics in the new building. The goal was to create a self-contained, friendly environment that would be secure for the residents and staff in this neighborhood plagued by the vagaries of urban society. The shape of the building responds to the client's desire for proximity between the nursing stations. Floors are composed of two 36-bed nursing units that are further divided into 18-bed "neighborhoods," each with its own bathing, utility, and lounge areas. The design promotes a smaller-scale residential character, and permits the principal caregivers to provide a high level of individual attention to the residents while allowing the client to contain the cost of operations.

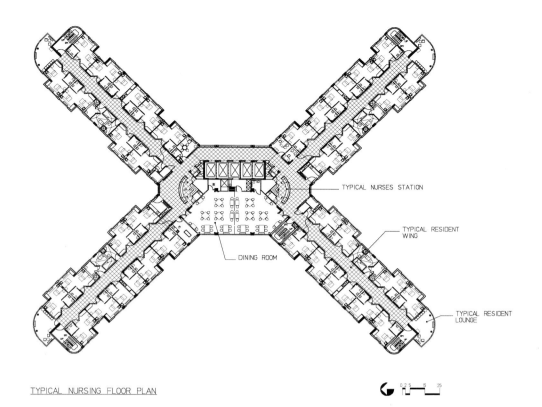

TYPICAL NURSES STATION

TYPICAL RESIDENT
WING

DINING ROOM

TYPICAL RESIDENT
LOUNGE

TYPICAL NURSING FLOOR PLAN

Credits (continued)

*Exterior, Insulation, and Finishing
System Consultant*

Williams Building Diagnostics, Inc.
Maple Glen, Pennsylvania

Food Service Consultants

JSR Consultants
Atlanta, Georgia

Construction Manager

Gotham Construction Corporation
New York, New York

Photographer

Peter Mauss/Esto Photographics
Mamaroneck, New York

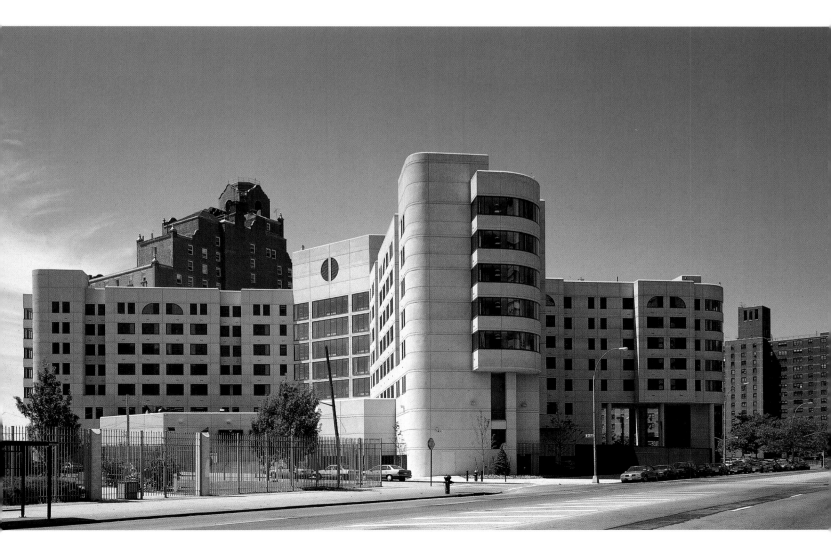

Sea Mar Intergenerational Community Care Center

Seattle, Washington

Owner
Sea Mar Community Health
Centers, Incorporated

Data
Type of Facility
Intergenerational skilled-nursing
facility

Context
Freestanding

Type of Construction
New

Area of Building
54,400 GSF

Cost of Construction
$8,198,800

Cost of Medical Equipment
$707,200

Status of Project
Completed September 1994

Credits
Architect
Donald I. King Architects, P.S.
1700 Bellevue Avenue, Suite 100
Seattle, Washington 98122

Associate Architect
Cornerstone Architectural Group
1904 Third Avenue, Suite 220
Seattle, Washington 98101

Structural Engineer
CT Engineering
Seattle, Washington

Mechanical Engineer
Sider and Byers
Seattle, Washington

Electrical Engineer
Casne Engineering
Seattle, Washington

Civil Engineer
Anne Symonds & Associates
Seattle, Washington

Landscape Architect
The Berger Partnership
Seattle, Washington

Long-Term Care Design Consultant
C. David Fey
Seattle, Washington

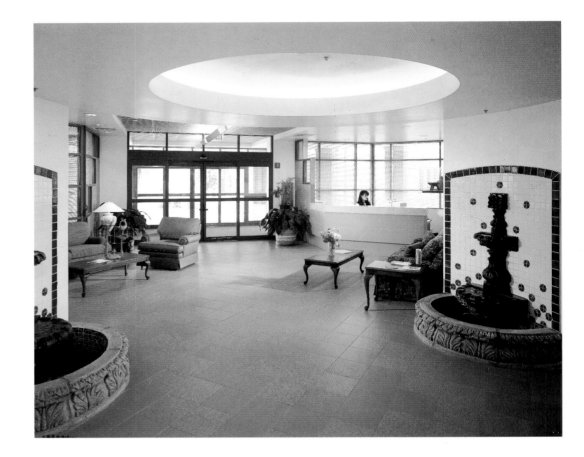

ARCHITECT'S STATEMENT

This 100-bed skilled-nursing facility and child development center for up to 90 children serves a predominantly low-income, Latino population. The design process involved the community directly in developing an intergenerational facility that would encourage families to visit; support the activities of both children and elders; and maximize the independence, privacy, and quality of life of its residents.

The center derives much of its design character from Mayan and Latin-American roots, with strong banded ornamentation, sloping parapets, crisp square window punches, and defined base. The interior is characterized by a hacienda courtyard lobby with fountains, skylights, decorative ceramics, and traditional home-style furnishings in the rich colors of the Latino culture. One-third of the child care program is housed in the skilled-nursing facility, encouraging intergenerational exchange. The child development center is designed with a skylit central commons surrounded by infant, early toddler, toddler, and preschool spaces.

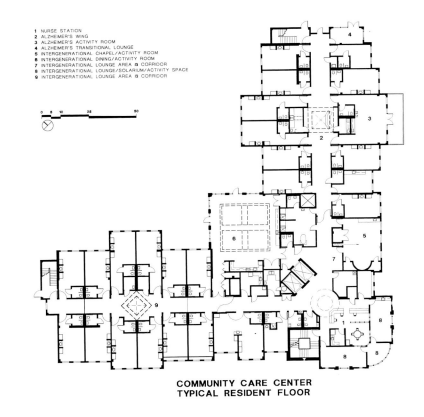

1 NURSE STATION
2 ALZHEIMER'S WING
3 ALZHEIMER'S ACTIVITY ROOM
4 ALZHEIMER'S TRANSITIONAL LOUNGE
5 INTERGENERATIONAL CHAPEL/ACTIVITY ROOM
6 INTERGENERATIONAL DINING/ACTIVITY ROOM
7 INTERGENERATIONAL LOUNGE AREA @ CORRIDOR
8 INTERGENERATIONAL LOUNGE/SOLARIUM/ACTIVITY SPACE
9 INTERGENERATIONAL LOUNGE AREA @ CORRIDOR

**COMMUNITY CARE CENTER
TYPICAL RESIDENT FLOOR**

Credits (continued)

*Child Care and Intergenerational
Design Consultant*

Bridgings Architects
Seattle, Washington

Contractor

Sellen Construction
Seattle, Washington

Photographers

Paris Yannis
Seattle, Washington

Steve Keating
Seattle, Washington

Michael Baum
Wauna, Washington

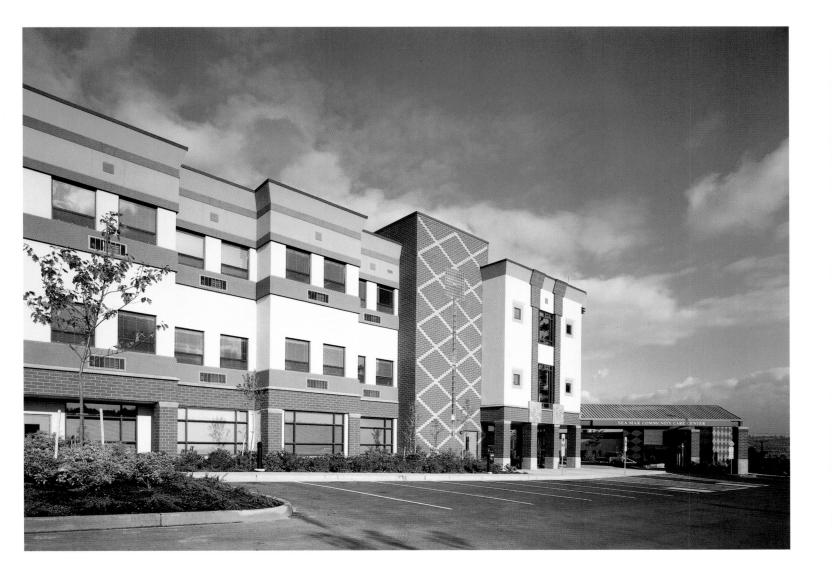

Fountain Court Nursing Center

Baton Rouge, Louisiana

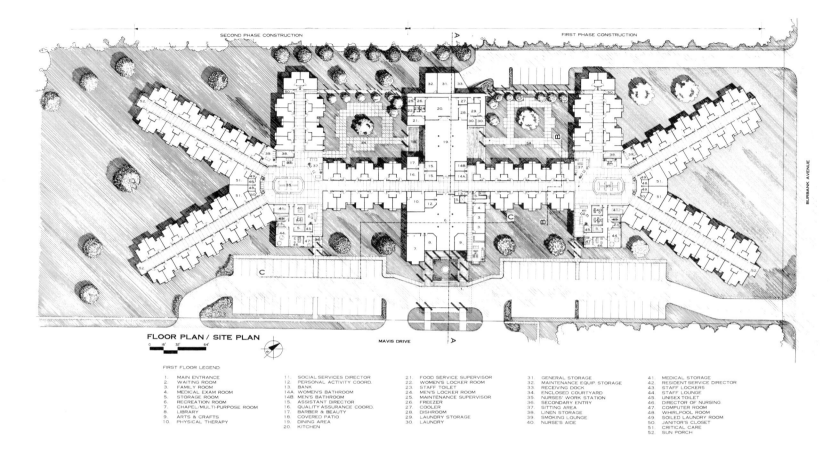

FLOOR PLAN / SITE PLAN

FIRST FLOOR LEGEND:

1. MAIN ENTRANCE	11. SOCIAL SERVICES DIRECTOR	21. FOOD SERVICE SUPERVISOR	31. GENERAL STORAGE	41. MEDICAL STORAGE
2. WAITING ROOM	12. PERSONAL ACTIVITY COORD.	22. WOMEN'S LOCKER ROOM	32. MAINTENANCE EQUIP. STORAGE	42. RESIDENT SERVICE DIRECTOR
3. FAMILY ROOM	13. BANK	23. STAFF TOILET	33. RECEIVING DOCK	43. STAFF LOCKERS
4. MEDICAL EXAM ROOM	14A. WOMEN'S BATHROOM	24. MEN'S LOCKER ROOM	34. ENCLOSED COURTYARD	44. STAFF LOUNGE
5. STORAGE ROOM	14B. MEN'S BATHROOM	25. MAINTENANCE SUPERVISOR	35. NURSES' WORK STATION	45. UNISEX TOILET
6. RECREATION ROOM	15. ASSISTANT DIRECTOR	26. FREEZER	36. SECONDARY ENTRY	46. DIRECTOR OF NURSING
7. CHAPEL/MULTI-PURPOSE ROOM	16. QUALITY ASSURANCE COORD.	27. COOLER	37. SITTING AREA	47. COMPUTER ROOM
8. LIBRARY	17. BARBER & BEAUTY	28. DISHROOM	38. LINEN STORAGE	48. WHIRLPOOL ROOM
9. ARTS & CRAFTS	18. COVERED PATIO	29. LAUNDRY STORAGE	39. SMOKING LOUNGE	49. SOILED LAUNDRY ROOM
10. PHYSICAL THERAPY	19. DINING AREA	30. LAUNDRY	40. NURSE'S AIDE	50. JANITOR'S CLOSET
	20. KITCHEN			51. CRITICAL CARE
				52. SUN PORCH

ARCHITECT'S STATEMENT

Located on the outskirts of a medium-sized southern city, this 250-bed facility is designed to furnish complete living and nursing facilities for elderly residents. The large central house includes major social activities, resident services, and dining. Administrative services are on the mezzanine level with views over major activity spaces. Resident bedrooms are designed to provide personal space with individual windows. This is supplemented with sunrooms at each wing, interior sitting areas at each nursing center, and exterior access to two controlled, enclosed garden patios.

The site is a former pecan orchard retaining specimen trees. The architecture recalls the traditional sloped sheltering rooflines and attics of the local vernacular architecture in all-fireproof materials.

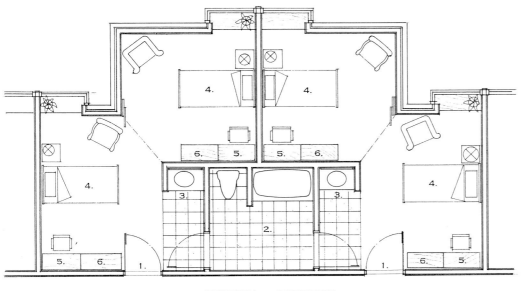

CENTRAL CORRIDOR

TYPICAL RESIDENT SUITE

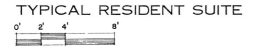

0'   2'   4'   8'

LEGEND
1. ENTRY
2. BATHROOM
3. LAVATORY
4. BED
5. DESK
6. WARDROBE CLOSET

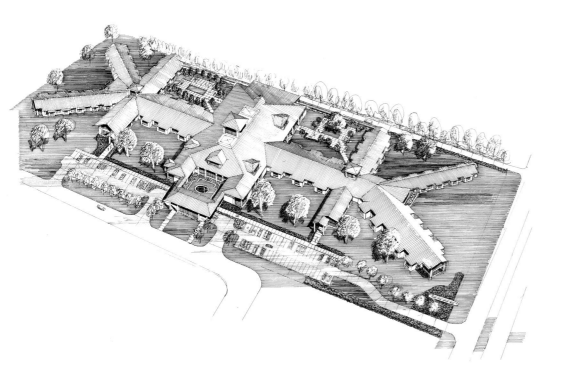

Owner
D&W Health Services, Inc.

Data

Type of Facility
Long-term residential health care facility

Context
Freestanding

Type of Construction
New

Area of Building
80,836 GSF

Cost of Construction
$4,850,160

Cost of Medical Equipment
$600,000

Status of Project
Estimated date of completion:
November 1996

Credits

Architect
John Desmond & Associates
Architects/Planners
703 Laurel Street
Baton Rouge, Louisiana 70802

Structural Engineer
McKee & Deville Consulting
Engineers
Baton Rouge, Louisiana

Mechanical Engineer
Mayers & Associates
Baton Rouge, Louisiana

Electrical Engineer
Daniel T. Calongne & Associates
Baton Rouge, Louisiana

Contractor
Not yet awarded

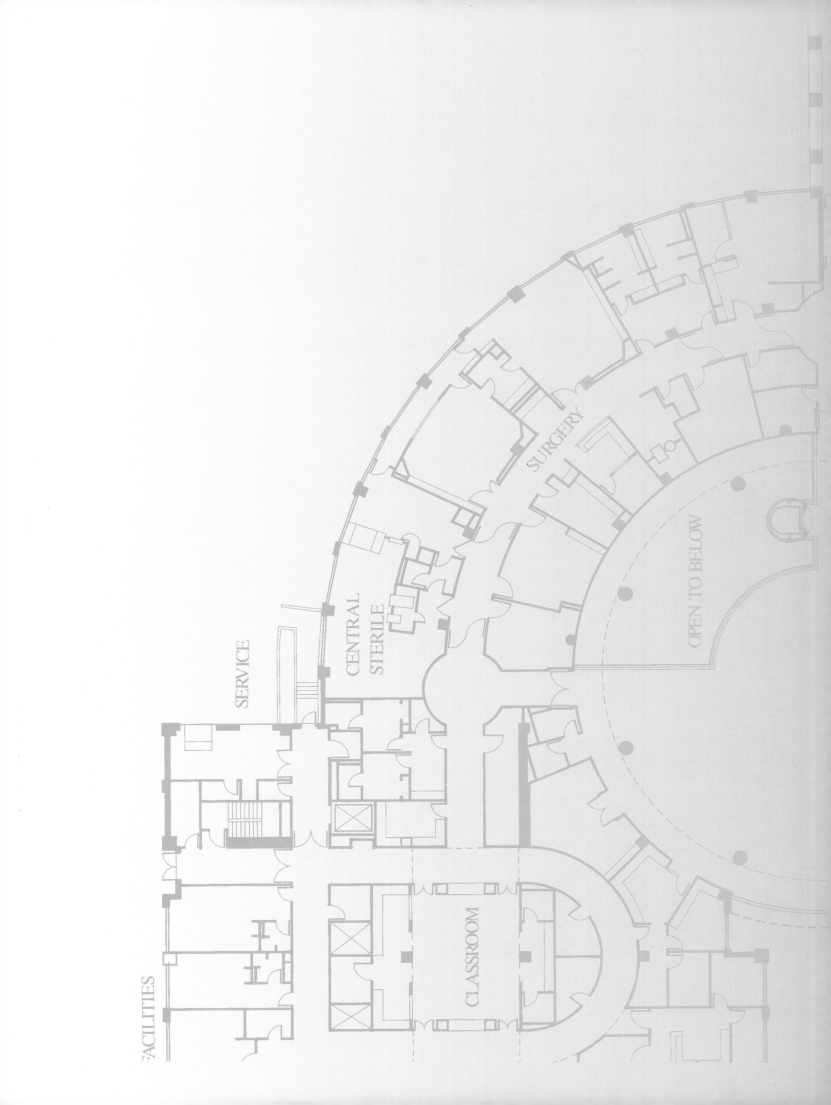

FACILITIES

SERVICE

CENTRAL
STERILE

SURGERY

CLASSROOM

OPEN TO BELOW

Pediatric Facilities

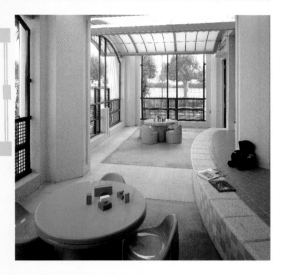

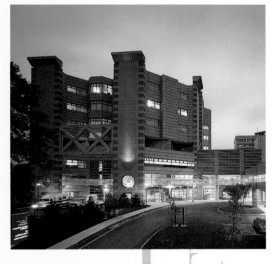

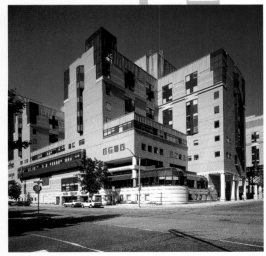

The Atrium at the Hospital for Sick Children

Toronto, Ontario, Canada

Owner
The Hospital for Sick Children
Toronto, Ontario, Canada

Data

Type of Facility
Addition to existing pediatric
hospital

Context
Hospital-based (572 beds)

Type of Construction
New

Area of Building
790,650 GSF (hospital building)
410,170 GSF (below-grade parking)

Cost of Construction
170,000,000 Canadian
($155,500,000 hospital building;
$14,500,000 parking)

Cost of Medical Equipment
$20,000,000 Canadian

Status of Project
Completed January 1993

Credits

Architect
Zeidler Roberts
Partnership/Architects
315 Queen Street West
Toronto, Ontario, Canada M5V 2X2

Associate Architect
Karlsberger & Associates Inc.
(hospital consultant)
99 East Main Street
Columbus, Ohio 43215

Structural Engineer
Carruthers & Wallace Ltd.
Toronto, Ontario

Mechanical/Electrical Engineer
Rybka, Smith & Ginsler Ltd.
Toronto, Ontario

Food Services Consultant
Cini-Little International Ltd.
Toronto, Ontario

Cost Consultant
Hanscomb Consultants Inc.
Toronto, Ontario

Code Consultant
Larden Muniak Consulting, Inc.
Toronto, Ontario

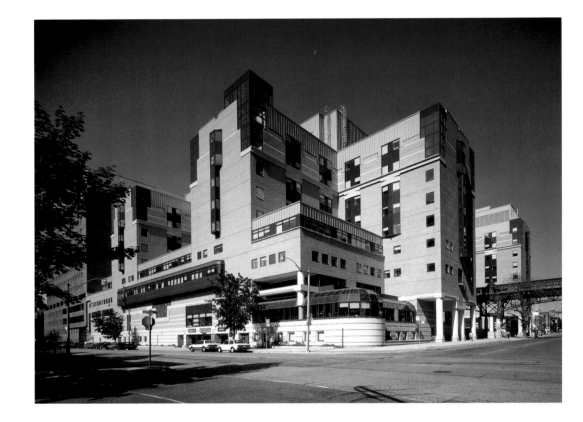

ARCHITECT'S STATEMENT

Through a series of additions made over the years, this world-famous pediatric hospital had crowded itself onto a tight downtown site. It was necessary to integrate existing facilities with new facilities, both functionally and visually. The program called for placement of the hospital's most urgent needs into a new structure, freeing most of the existing buildings for future services. The new eight-level building integrates and completes a previously undefined inner-city building block.

The new patient tower addition is organized around a large double atrium. In addition to improving orientation, the atria landscaping and artwork provide a positive healing environment. To respond to the emotional needs of sick children, single-patient rooms contain sofa beds for use by parents. Materials and colors were selected for their timeless quality and cross-cultural appeal.

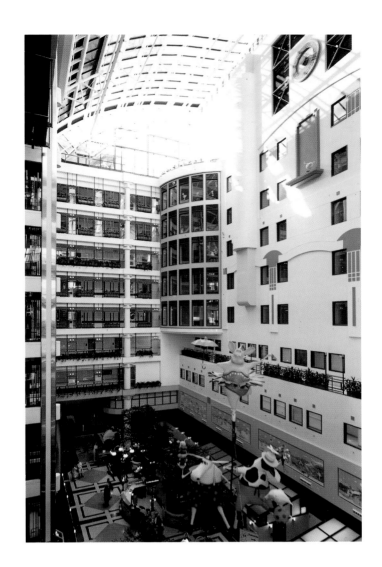

Credits (continued)
Contractors
Pigott Construction Ltd.
(superstructure)
Toronto, Ontario

Eastern Construction Co. Ltd.
(substructure)
Toronto, Ontario

Photographers
Balthazar Korab Ltd.
Troy, Michigan

Lenscape
Toronto, Ontario

Steven Evans Photography Inc.
Toronto, Ontario

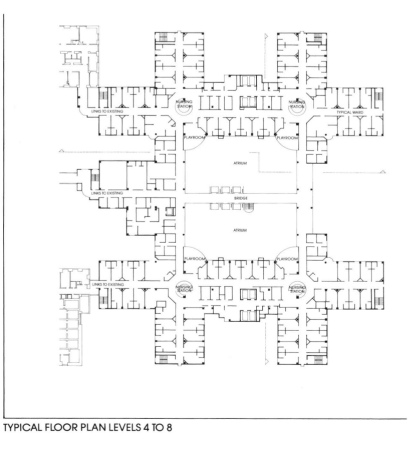

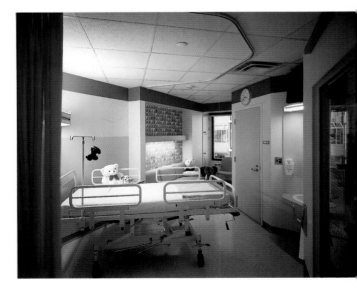

TYPICAL FLOOR PLAN LEVELS 4 TO 8

Children's National Medical Center/Children's Research Institute

Washington, D.C.

Owner
Children's National Medical Center

Data
Type of Facility
Rooftop addition to clinical research laboratory

Context
Hospital-based: no beds

Type of Construction
New

Area of Building
55,000 GSF

Cost of Construction
$8,360,000

Cost of Medical Equipment
$90,000

Status of Project
Completed January 1995

Credits
Architect
Ellerbe Becket
1875 Connecticut Avenue, N.W.
Suite 600
Washington, D.C. 20009

Structural Engineer
Simistova, Kehnumui & Associates
Rockville, Maryland

Mechanical/Electrical Engineer
Smith Seckman Reid, Inc.
Nashville, Tennessee

Laboratory Consultant
Earl Walls Associate
San Diego, California

Contractor
The George Hyman Construction Company
Bethesda, Maryland

Photographer
Maxwell MacKenzie
Washington, D.C.

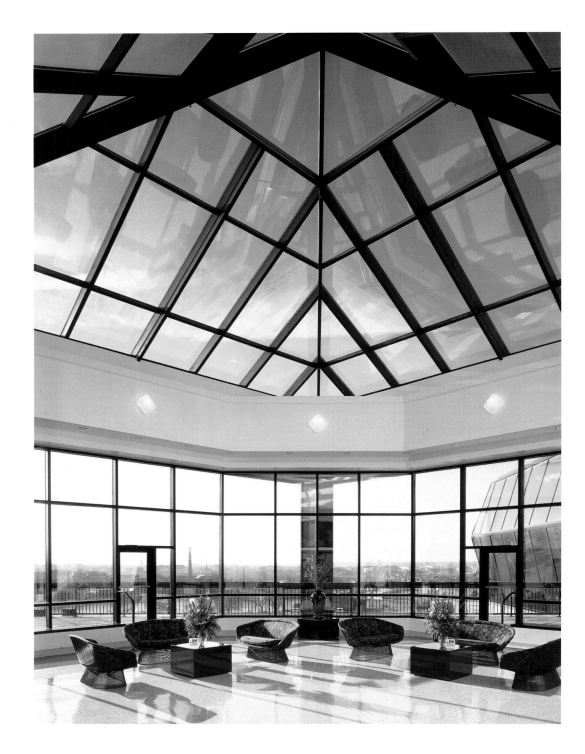

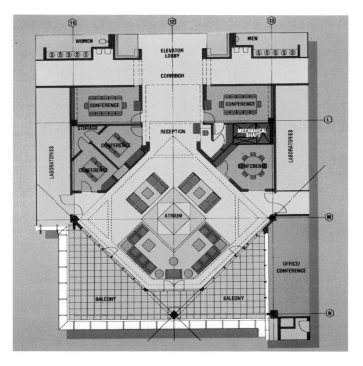

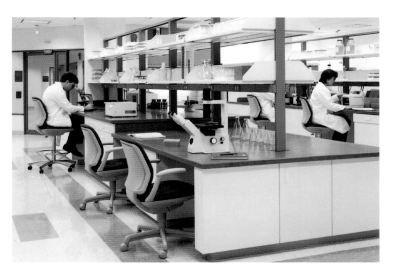

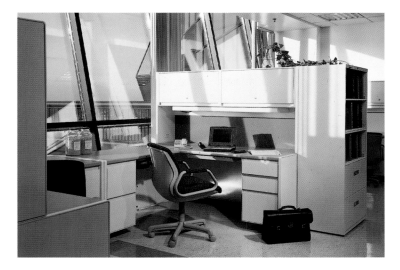

ARCHITECT'S STATEMENT

Children's National Medical Center created a research institute to bring critical medical research to the bedside and ambulatory environment, in order to address the urgent health care needs of children today. The desire for proximity to the treatment programs and the lack of adjacent available land led to the Children's Research Institute, a rooftop clinical lab addition, combining both shelled and fit-out space for six important centers of research. A skylit central atrium provides appropriate conference and reception space for grant development and multidisciplined consultation. An interstitial service deck and standardized lab benches with custom-fitted cabinetry maximize planning flexibility.

Hasbro Children's Hospital at Rhode Island Hospital

Providence, Rhode Island

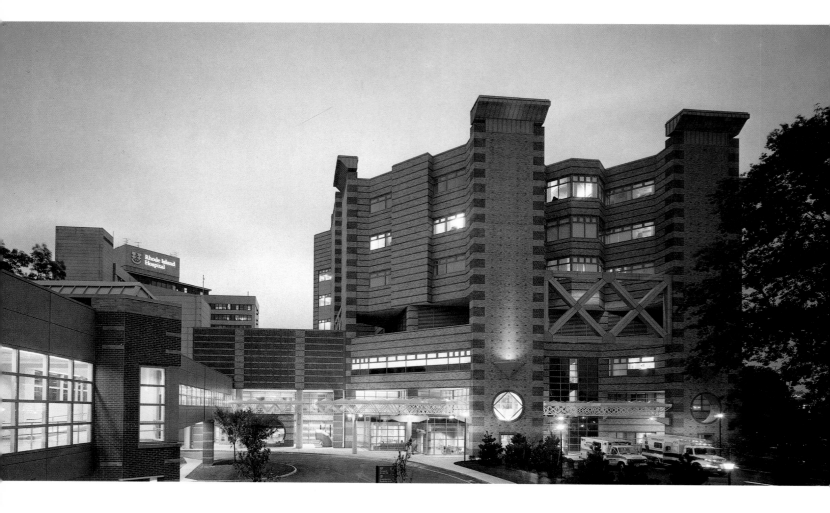

A R C H I T E C T ' S   S T A T E M E N T

Designed from the ground up as a special place for children, Hasbro Children's Hospital integrates pediatric diagnostic and treatment functions with patient beds in a new building, part of a long-range facilities plan. Program elements include a 16-bed intensive care unit, physical therapy, and three 24-bed patient care units designated by age. Surgery, emergency, and radiology suites are near adult services to provide flexibility. A double-height lobby links two major hospital entrances and features a playhouse, fountain, aquarium, and gift shop. At ground level, the building houses a pediatric clinic with space for primary and adolescent care, specialty, and cancer units.

Clustering the inpatient units provides proximity for care-giver, child, and family. It also permits patients with differing nursing needs to be grouped together and allows ready renovation to intensive care in the future. Each of the three floors is a "neighborhood" for 24 children and their families, with playrooms, an activity area, and classrooms with closed-circuit television. Among the many murals and sculptures, a rough-hewn granite fountain with interactive controls is in the lobby, and 11,000 ceramic tiles crafted by local school children are featured in corridors and nurses' stations.

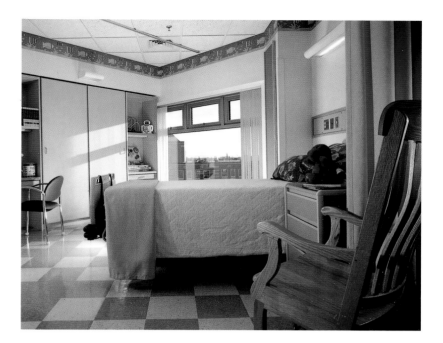

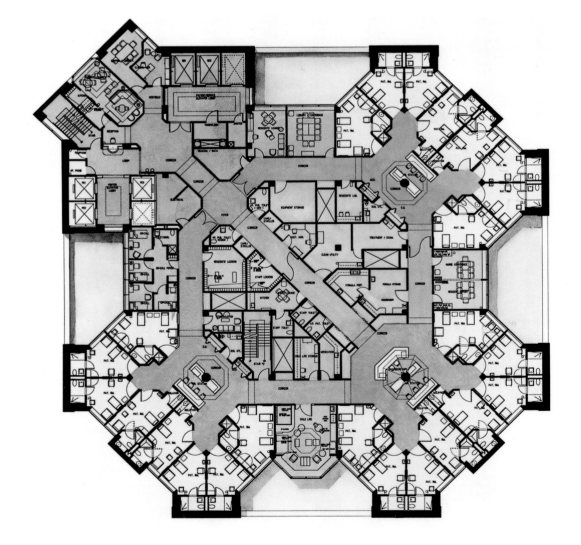

O w n e r
Rhode Island Hospital

D a t a

Type of Facility
Pediatric hospital

Context
Hospital-based: 87 beds

Type of Construction
New

Area of Building
190,205 GSF

Cost of Construction
$38,136,000

Cost of Medical Equipment
$3,447,000

Status of Project
Completed 1994

C r e d i t s

Architect
Shepley Bulfinch Richardson and Abbott
40 Broad Street
Boston, Massachusetts 02109

Structural Engineer
Zaldastani Associates
Boston, Massachusetts

Mechanical/Electrical Engineer
BR+A Consulting Engineers
Boston, Massachusetts

Landscape Architect
Walker-Kluesing Design Group
Boston, Massachusetts

Furnishings Consultant
Rosalyn Cama Interior Design Associates
New Haven, Connecticut

Equipment Consultant
Charles Heinemann Associates, Inc.
Eden Prairie, Minnesota

Contractor
Gilbane Building Company
Providence, Rhode Island

Photographers
Robert Miller
Reston, Virginia

Jean Smith
Cambridge, Massachusetts

The Don Imus-WFAN Pediatric Center for Tomorrow's Children at Hackensack Medical Center

Hackensack, New Jersey

Owner
Hackensack Medical Center

Data
Type of Facility
Ambulatory care center for children

Context
Freestanding

Type of Construction
New

Area of Building
90,000 GSF

Cost of Construction
$17,899,490

Cost of Medical Equipment
$640,253

Status of Project
Completed June 1994

Credits
Architect
Perkins & Will
One Park Avenue, 19th Floor
New York, New York 10016

Structural Engineer
Alfred Selnick, P.E., P.C.
New York, New York

Mechanical/Electrical Engineer
Goldman Copeland Associates, P.C.
New York, New York

Elevator Consultant
Calvin L. Kort
Glen Rock, New Jersey

Contractor
William Blanchard Construction
Springfield, New Jersey

Photographer
Jeff Goldberg at Esto
Photographics
Mamaroneck, New York

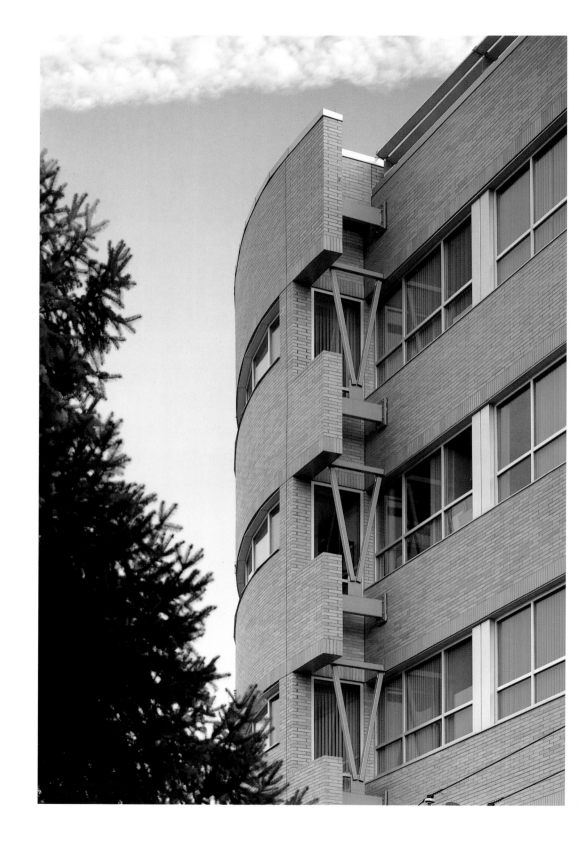

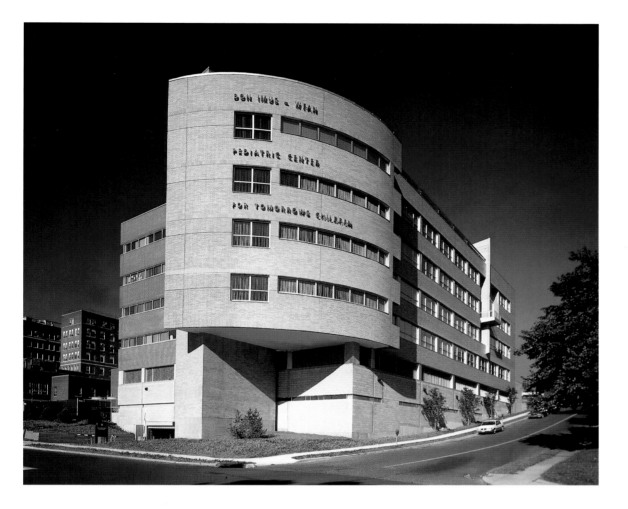

Designed to create a colorful, humane environment for hundreds of children and their parents each year, the Don Imus-WFAN Pediatric Center for Tomorrow's Children at Hackensack Medical Center is the largest facility providing sophisticated outpatient cancer care for children in the eastern United States.

The 90,000-square-foot, four-story facility is divided into two distinct wings, with a new entrance atrium opening the medical campus and orienting patients and visitors to all levels. Office and meeting spaces are located in the north wing, while the exam and treatment areas of the children's cancer center and pediatric behavioral medicine programs are in the south wing, linked to the hospital via a second-story bridge.

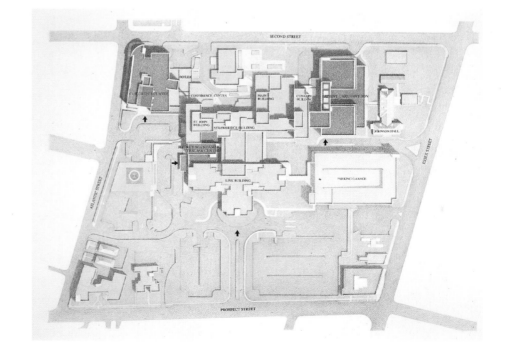

Loma Linda University Medical Center Children's Hospital

Loma Linda, California

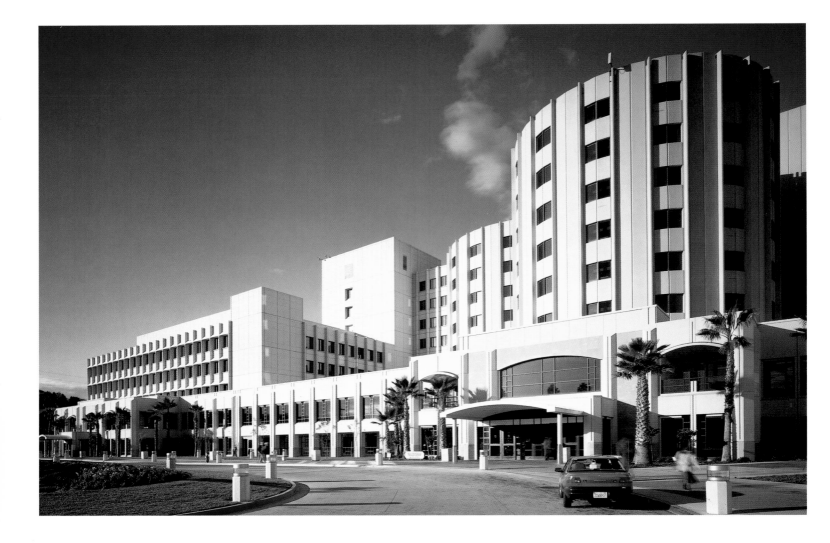

ARCHITECT'S STATEMENT

ARCHITECT'S STATEMENT

Children's Hospital is the infill of a major addition to the medical center. The purpose of the project was to consolidate the Children's Services portion of this major medical center in one location. The new Children's Hospital infill project took as its design theme one of "discovery." It is intended to amuse the child and provide a means for the parent to engage the child's imagination and sense of wonder in a place that can be very frightening. It is also intended to educate the child and the parent about aspects of that child's world.

The patient rooms are clustered, with support services concentrated at the nurse's fingertips. Each nurses' station has a direct view of eight patient beds.

The work areas are separated from the patient care areas. Patient rooms consist of one-bed rooms, two-bed rooms, and isolation rooms. All rooms in the new Children's Hospital infill are classified as intensive care units.

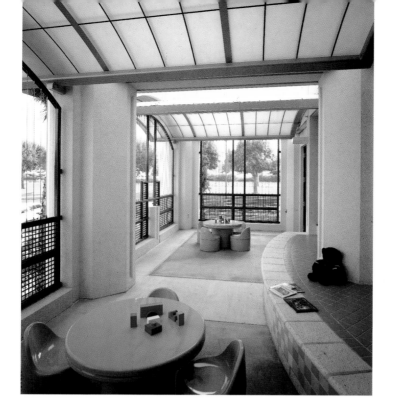

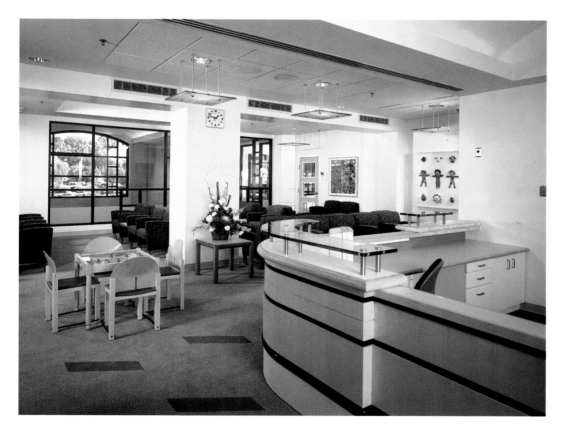

O w n e r
  Loma Linda University Medical
  Center Adventist Health Systems

D a t a
  Type of Facility
  Children's Hospital

  Context
  Hospital-based: 66 beds

  Type of Construction
  New

  Area of Building
  96,513 GSF

  Cost of Construction
  $13,606,767

  Cost of Medical Equipment
  $6,700,000

  Status of Project
  Completed December 1993

C r e d i t s
  Architect
  NBBJ
  130 Sutter Street, 2nd Street
  San Francisco, California 94104

  Structural Engineer
  Skilling Ward Magnusson Barkshire
  Seattle, Washington

  Mechanical Engineer
  Notkin Engineering
  Seattle Washington

  Electrical Engineer
  Sparling & Associates
  Seattle, Washington

  Acoustical Consultant
  Towne Richards Chaudiere
  Seattle, Washington

  Art Consultant
  American Art Resources
  Houston, Texas

  Contractor
  McCarthy Construction
  Irvine, California

  Photographer
  Hewitt/Garrison Photography
  San Diego, California

Shriners Hospitals for Crippled Children, Intermountain Unit

Salt Lake City, Utah

Owner

Shriners Hospitals for Crippled
Children

Data

Type of Facility

Pediatric orthopedic hospital

Context

Hospital-based: 40 beds

Type of Construction

New

Area of Building

110,000 GSF

Cost of Construction

Not available

Cost of Medical Equipment

Not available

Status of Project

Estimated completion date:
September 1995

Credits

Architect

Odell Associates Inc.
129 West Trade Street
Charlotte, North Carolina 28202

*Structural Engineer/Mechanical/
Electrical Engineer*

Odell Associates Inc.
Charlotte, North Carolina

Consulting Structural/Seismic Engineer

EQE International
San Francisco, California

Food Service

Foodesign
Charlotte, North Carolina

Interior Design

Odell Associates Inc.
Charlotte, North Carolina

Construction Manager

Barton Malow Company
Southfield, Michigan

Photographer

Tim Buchman
Charlotte, North Carolina

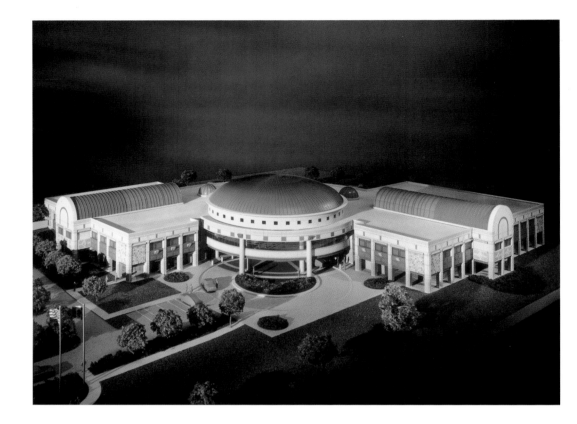

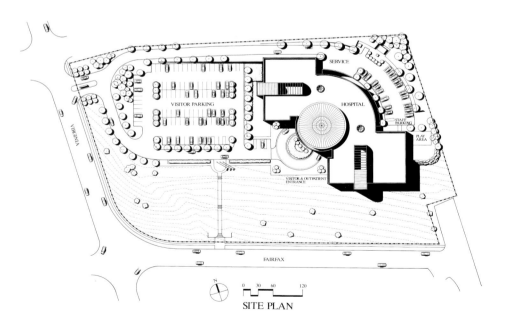

SITE PLAN

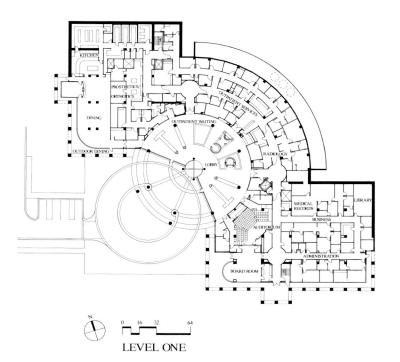

LEVEL ONE

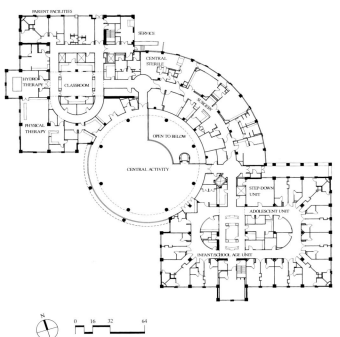

LEVEL TWO

ARCHITECT'S STATEMENT

The proposed project provides a replacement hospital for the existing facility constructed in the early 1950s. Natural materials are featured on the new building's exterior. Native Utah limestone and red sandstone are selected as the cladding for the concrete structure. Decorative precast concrete panels serve as spandrels below the second-level windows. A domed central activity space on the second level provides the facility with its most striking visual element. All inpatient traffic passes through this lofty space. The exterior windows are focused to the southwest to encompass a sweeping vista of downtown Salt Lake City and the mountains beyond.

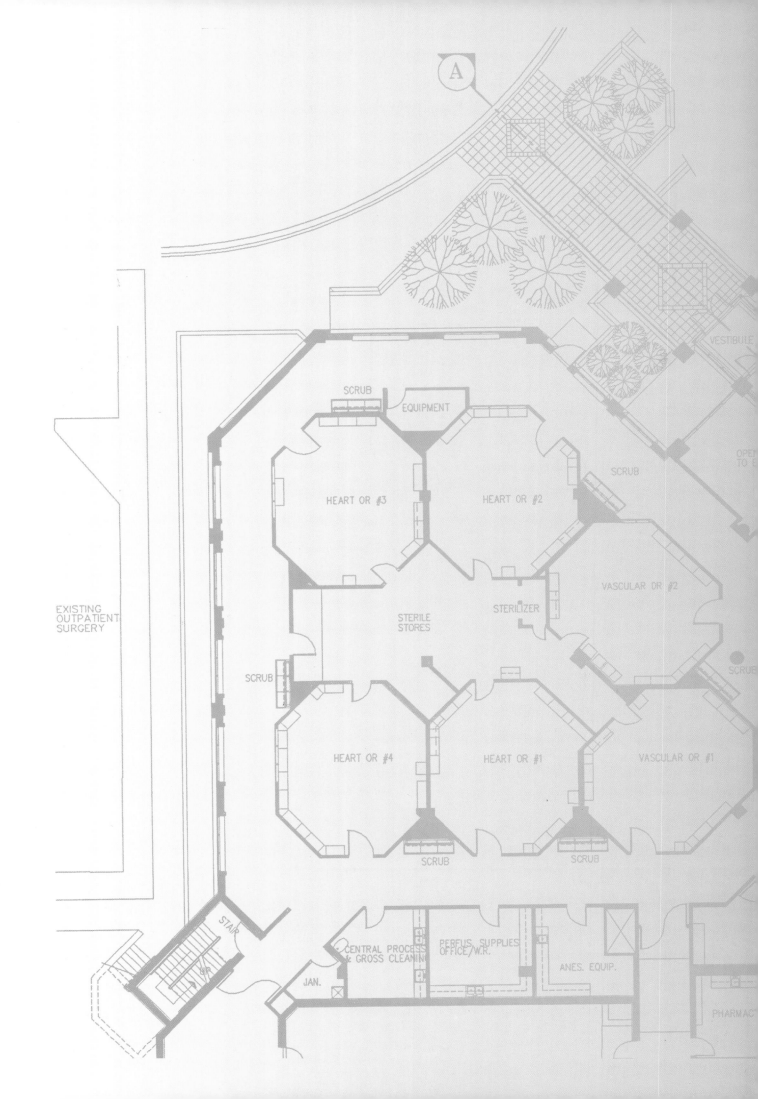

Specialty Facilities

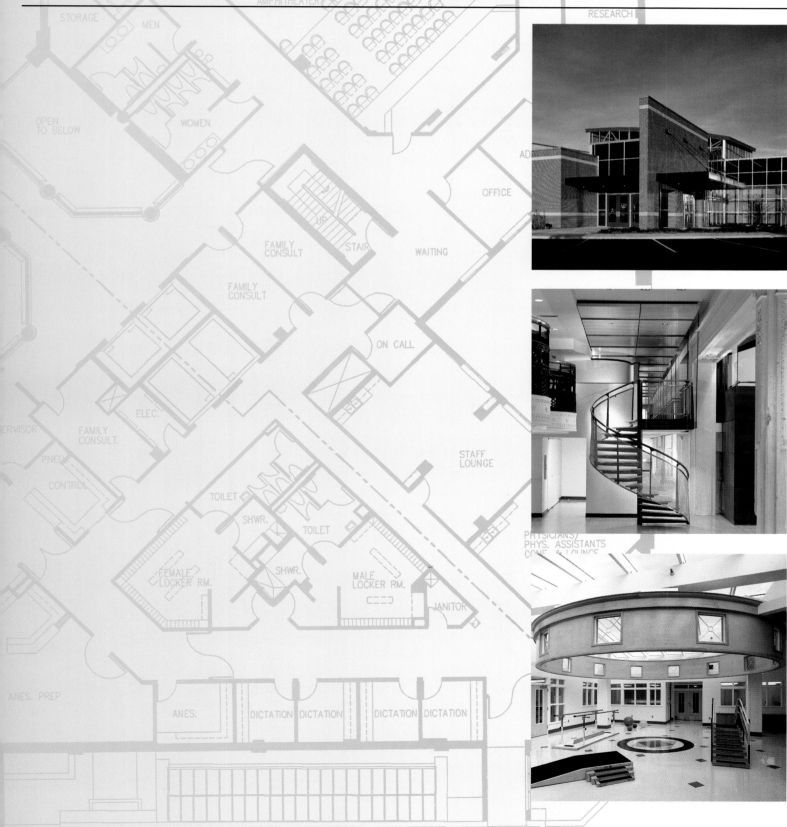

La Palestra Center for Preventative Medicine

New York, New York

Citation

This facility is a unique blend of old and new, carefully inserting new functions and forms into the shelled relic of a 1920s-era grand ballroom in Manhattan. The careful execution and restraint of this project are remarkable. Detailing of the new elements such as ceiling, skylighting, steel wall structures, and finishes is very elegantly handled, indicating an intentional respect for the original facility. The fabric of the original ballroom is left as is, dramatically lit and preserved as opposed to being restored or adapted. The development of public spaces is refined, warm, and richly textured. The mission of this center to enrich both the body and mind is achieved quite capably.

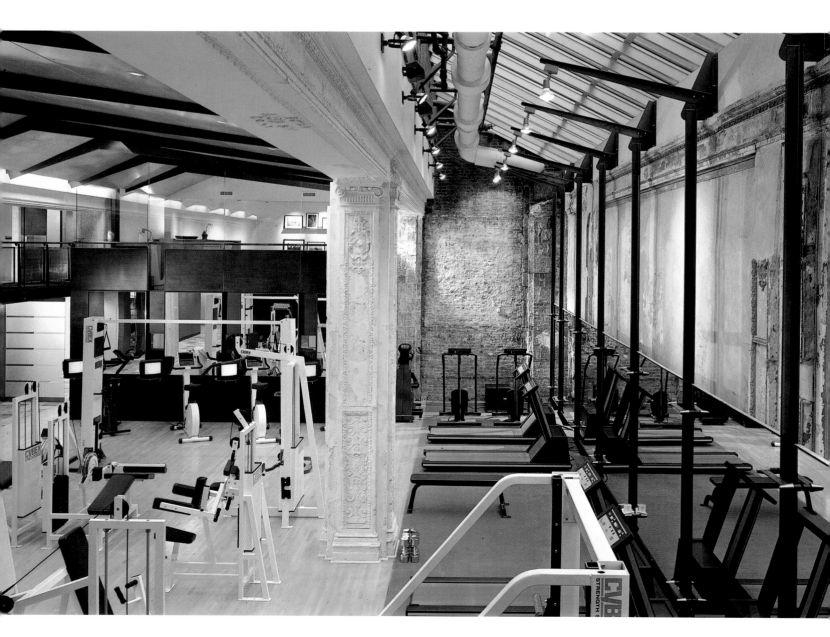

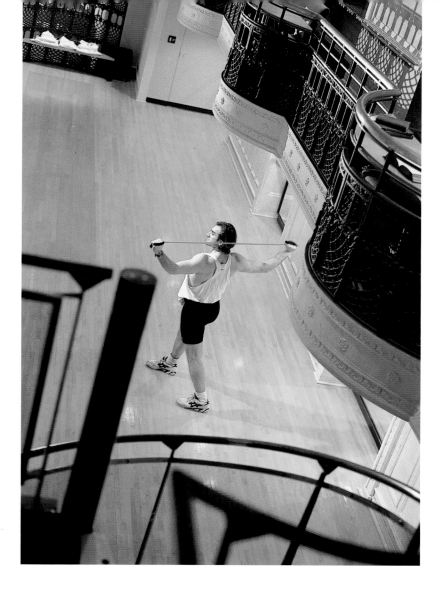

Owner
Pasquale Manocchia

Data

Type of Facility
Preventive medicine and physical
therapy

Context
Freestanding

Type of Construction
Renovation

Area of Building
16,000 GSF

Cost of Construction
$1,900,000

Cost of Medical Equipment
$350,000

Status of Project
Completed March 1995

Credits

Architect
HLW International LLP
115 Fifth Avenue
New York, New York 10003

Interior Designer
HLW International LLP

*Structural/Mechanical/Electrical
Engineer*
HLW International LLP
New York, New York

Contractor
Foster Haimes Construction
Partnership
New York, New York

Photographers
Scott Frances/Esto Photography
Mamaroneck, New York

Peter Paige
Harrington Park, New Jersey

ARCHITECT'S STATEMENT

Located in a renovated space of a landmark ball-room, the facility offers prescribed diagnostic, thera-peutic, rehabilitative, and preventive cardiovascular and orthopedic medical services for improved health. Elegant forms and details converge in a dialogue of old and new, scale and texture, material and color. The space's original grandeur was recaptured by maintain-ing original columns, beams, and exterior walls and reconnecting the once-subdivided space. New ele-ments, such as the fully accessible mezzanine, ribbed wood ceiling, and a 150-foot skylight, were carefully inserted into the existing shell, reflecting the facility's combination of human and technological characteris-tics in its architectural form.

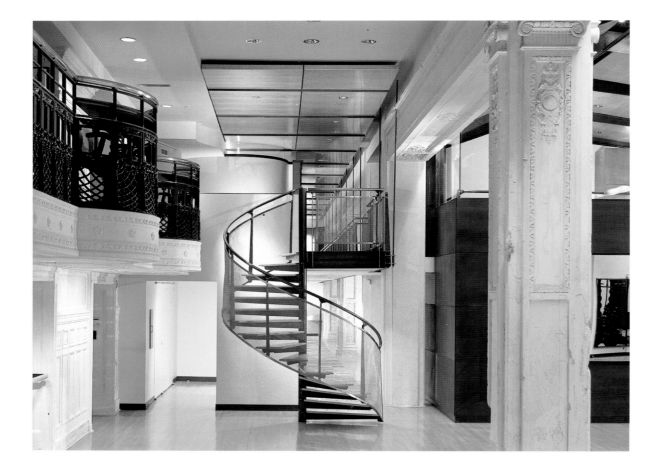

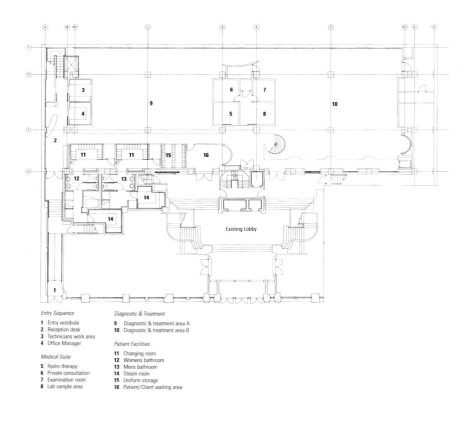

Entry Sequence

1 Entry vestibule
2 Reception desk
3 Technicians work area
4 Office Manager

Medical Suite

5 Hydro therapy
6 Private consultation
7 Examination room
8 Lab sample area

Diagnostic & Treatment

9 Diagnostic & treatment area A
10 Diagnostic & treatment area B

Patient Facilities

11 Changing room
12 Womens bathroom
13 Mens bathroom
14 Steam room
15 Uniform storage
16 Patient/Client waiting area

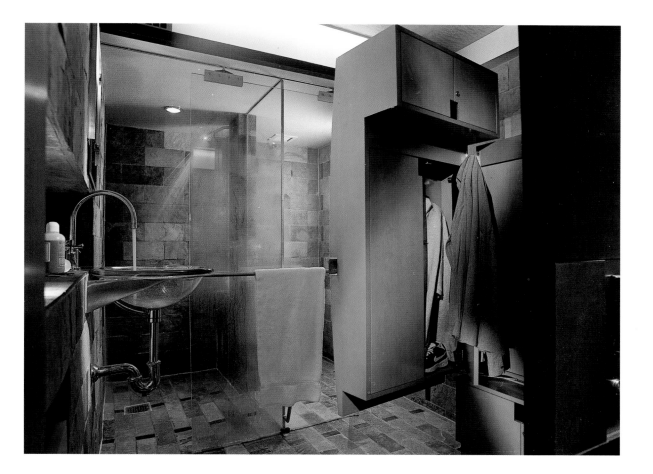

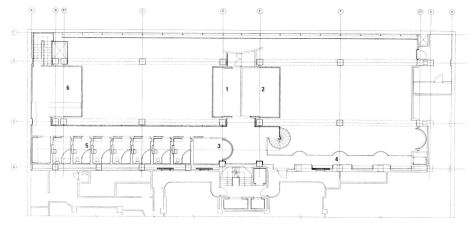

Mezzanine

1 Patient/Client consultation
2 Program directors office
3 Therapy room
4 Reference library
5 Private changing rooms
6 Patient/Client Lounge

Health Bridge Fitness Center

Crystal Lake, Illinois

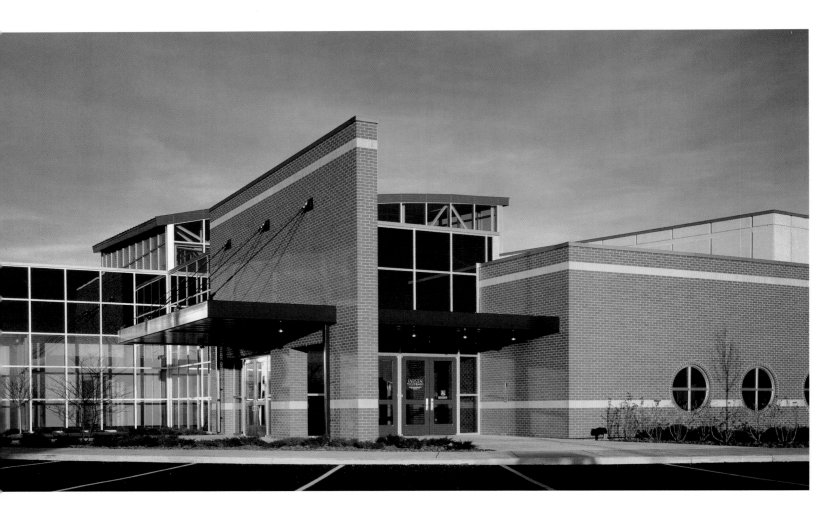

ARCHITECT'S STATEMENT

With the development of its health and fitness center, the hospital is delivering on its mission of wellness within the community. The facility features fitness, medical rehabilitation, and community education programs that emphasize preventive medicine and wellness services. This is the first building built at the hospital's satellite ambulatory campus and was completed—design through owner occupancy—within a period of 16 months and within budget.

The design was driven by the linear organization of functions defined by their massing. The lobby acts as a transitional element, with its curved roof monitor linking the clinical and community spaces to the massive fitness functions. While introducing natural light into the building core, the monitor also acts as a primary architectural expression of the exterior, which consists of brick, precast concrete, glass, and aluminum curtain wall.

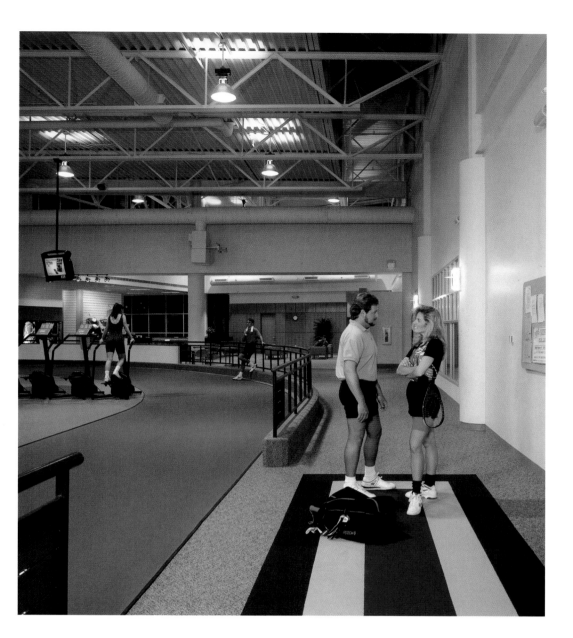

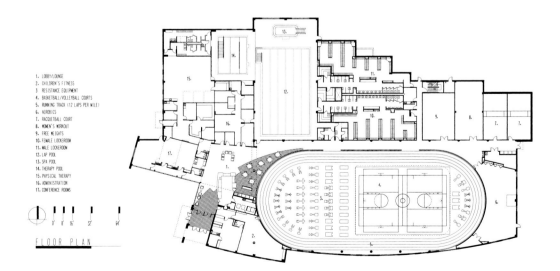

1. LOBBY/LOUNGE
2. CHILDREN'S FITNESS
3. RESISTANCE EQUIPMENT
4. BASKETBALL/VOLLEYBALL COURTS
5. RUNNING TRACK (12 LAPS PER MILE)
6. AEROBICS
7. RACQUETBALL COURT
8. WOMEN'S WORKOUT
9. FREE WEIGHTS
10. FEMALE LOCKEROOM
11. MALE LOCKEROOM
12. LAP POOL
13. SPA POOL
14. THERAPY POOL
15. PHYSICAL THERAPY
16. ADMINISTRATION
17. CONFERENCE ROOMS

0' 8' 16'   32'   64'

FLOOR PLAN

O w n e r
Northern Illinois Medical Center
Foundation

D a t a
Type of Facility
Hospital-based health
and wellness center

Context
Freestanding

Type of Construction
New

Area of Building
57,205 GSF

Cost of Construction
$5,330,000

Cost of Medical Equipment
$321,000

Status of Project
Completed December 1994

C r e d i t s
Architect
Phillips Swager Associates
3622 N. Knoxville Avenue
Peoria, Illinois 61603-1079

Consulting Architect
William Merci, Architect
1331 Sheridan Road
Wilmette, Illinois 60091

*Structural/Mechanical/Electrical
Engineer*
Phillips Swager Associates
Peoria, Illinois

Fitness Center Consultant
Hospital Fitness Corporation
Evanston, Illinois

Owner Representative
Morgan Construction
Consultants, Inc.
Chicago, Illinois

Contractor
W. B. Olson, Inc.
Northbrook, Illinois

Photographer
Barry Rustin Photography
Glenview, Illinois

The Catherine and Charles Owen Heart Center

Asheville, North Carolina

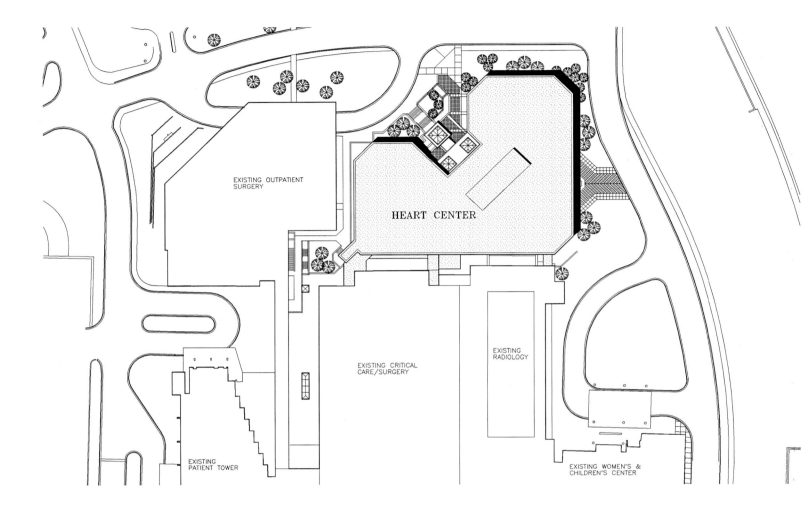

EXISTING OUTPATIENT
SURGERY

HEART CENTER

EXISTING CRITICAL
CARE/SURGERY

EXISTING
RADIOLOGY

EXISTING
PATIENT TOWER

EXISTING WOMEN'S &
CHILDREN'S CENTER

ARCHITECT'S STATEMENT

Program components of this five-story addition to the existing hospital include four open-heart surgery suites and two vascular surgery suites (also equipped for open-heart procedures), associated support functions, a four-bed recovery unit, 32-bed intensive care unit, 40-bed cardiovascular progressive-care unit for surgical patients, 40-bed medical cardiology unit, family waiting area, boardroom, 70-seat theater, and administrative space.

A small site and the need to link the addition to related levels in the existing hospital presented the major challenges in designing the building. The design solution identifies the building as one of the hospital's "Centers of Excellence" while harmonizing with other buildings on campus.

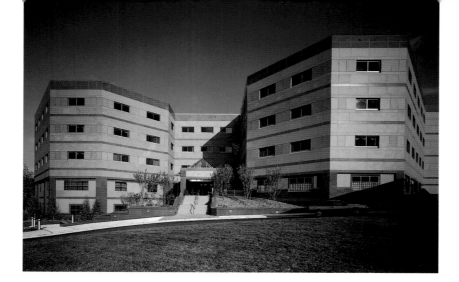

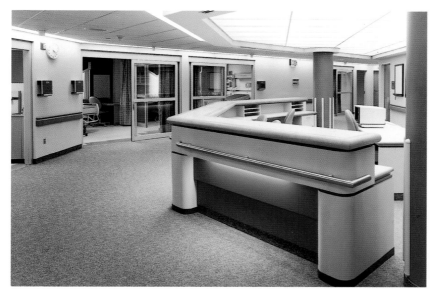

Owner
Memorial Mission Hospital, Inc.

Data
Type of Facility

Heart services (diagnosis, pacemakers and implantable defibrillators, electrophysiology, cardiovascular surgery, medical cardiology, pediatric cardiology)

Context

Hospital-based: 116 beds

Type of construction

New

Area of Building

125,000 GSF

Cost of Construction

Not available

Status of project

Completed April 1995

Credits
Architect

Padgett & Freeman Architects, P.A.
30 Choctaw Street
Asheville, North Carolina 28801

Structural Engineer

Sutton-Kennerly & Associates
Asheville, North Carolina

Mechanical Engineer

Mechanical Engineers, Inc.
Charlotte, North Carolina

Electrical Engineer

Reece, Noland & McElrath, Inc.
Waynesville, North Carolina

Landscape Architect

Heery International
Atlanta, Georgia

Contractor

McDevitt Street Bovis, Inc.
Charlotte, North Carolina

Photographer

J. Weiland
Asheville, North Carolina

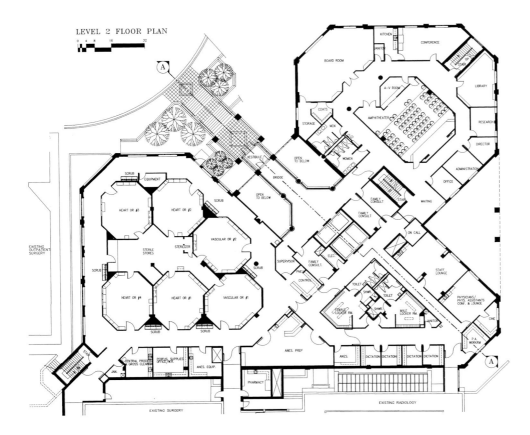

LEVEL 2 FLOOR PLAN

Sequoia Hospital Acute Care Rehabilitation Unit

Redwood City, California

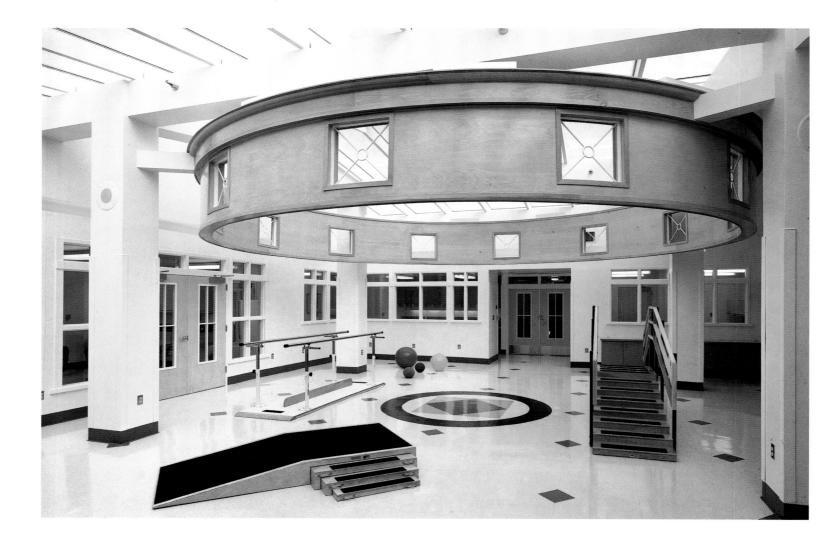

The design, which was constrained by the hospital's existing conditions, program, and budget requirements, supports the delivery of a broad range of care to patients of various acuities. It takes advantage of an existing courtyard to create a skylit gymnasium that is the focus of the unit's design and is used for active rehabilitation services. Ancillary rooms are oriented to provide a view of the gym. Reflecting the hospital's philosophy that the patient's physical environment lends itself to the healing process, the unit's interior design is cheerful and comfortable, using natural light, colors, finishes, and materials selected to make patients feel at ease.

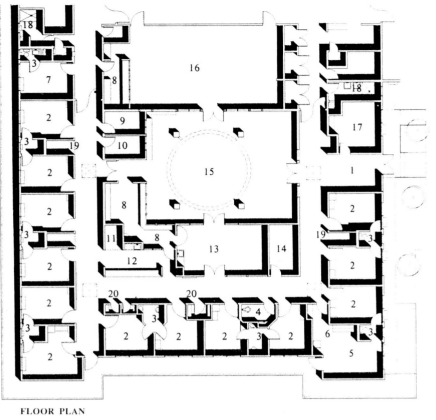

FLOOR PLAN

1	Lobby	11	File Storage
2	Patient Room	12	Nurse Station
3	Bathroom	13	Community Room
4	Visitor Bathroom	14	Speech Therapy
5	Transition Apartment	15	Occupational and Physical Therapy Gym
6	Kitchen	16	Dayroom
7	Exam Room	17	Conference Room
8	Therapist Chart Room	18	Shower
9	Medical Director	19	Linen Cart Storage
10	Program Director	20	Medical Supplies

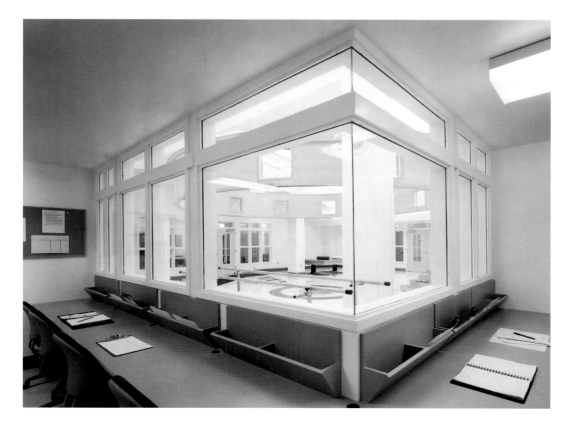

Owner
Sequoia Hospital District

Data

Type of Facility
Rehabilitation unit

Context
Hospital-based: 14 beds

Type of Construction
Renovation

Area of Building
3,700 GSF

Cost of Construction
$390,000

Cost of Medical Equipment
Not available

Status of Project
Completed July 1993

Credits

Architect
DES Architects + Engineers
399 Bradford Street
Redwood City, California 94063

Structural Engineer
DES Architects + Engineers
Redwood City, California

Mechanical/Electrical Engineer
S&H Engineers
San Francisco, California

Director of Program
Steven Allen
BAK Physical Therapy
Redwood City, California

Contractor
L&S Hallmark Construction
Sunnyvale, California

Photographer
Vittoria Visuals
San Francisco, California

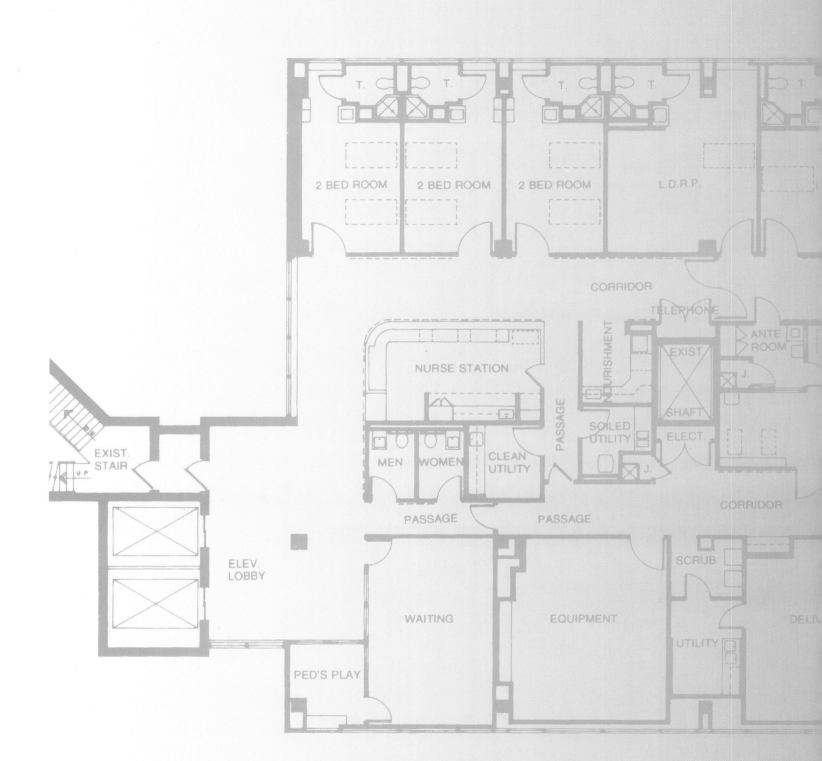

Women's Health Care Centers

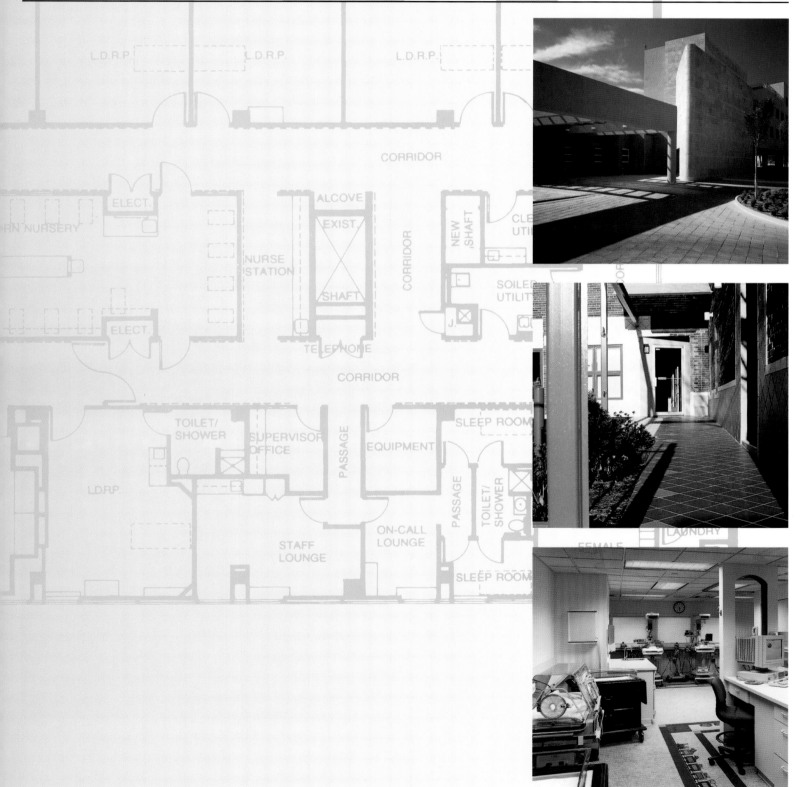

Mary's Center for Maternal & Child Care

Washington, D.C.

Citation

This modest project is successful at multiple levels. It rigorously evaluates existing site and building resources and skillfully deploys the program in a way that achieves logical functional accommodation with minimal modification of existing construction. It does so not only to control costs but also to achieve a design scale appropriate to the objective of providing primary care services in a familiar setting.

Through color selection and careful detailing, ordinary materials (paint, tile, fixture wiring) achieve a sparkling interior. Minimal exterior changes—window replacement, an elegant fence, and the use of color—unify the individual buildings that constitute the project and contribute a friendly community presence.

Before

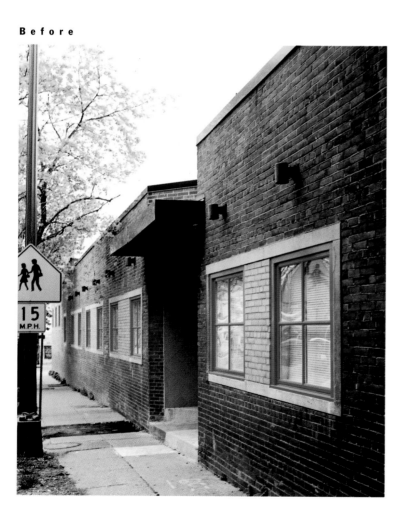

After

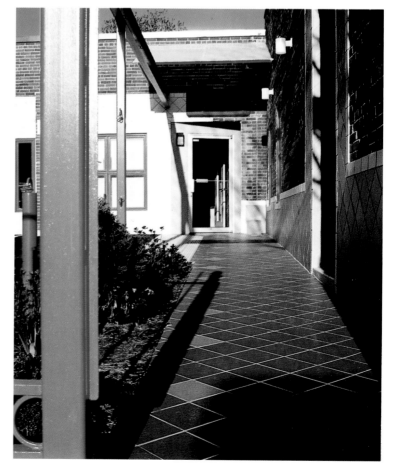

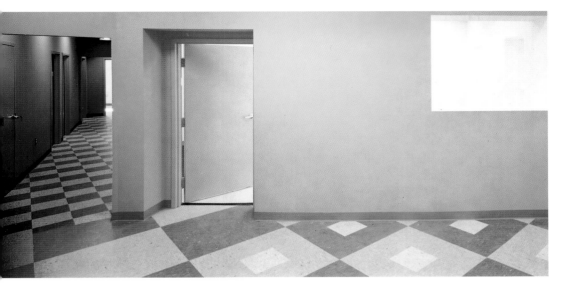

Owner
  Mary's Center for Maternal &
  Child Care, Inc.

Data
  Type of Facility
    Maternal and child care clinic

  Context
    Freestanding

  Type of Construction
    Renovation

  Area of Building
    6,900 GSF

  Cost of Construction
    $514,800

  Cost of Medical Equipment
    None

  Status of Project
    Completed January 1995

Credits
  Architect
    Robert Schwartz Associates
    Architects
    1811 18th Street, NW
    Washington, D.C. 20009

  Structural Engineer
    Cates Engineering
    Sterling, Virginia

  Mechanical/Electrical Engineer
    Petrossian Associates
    McLean, Virginia

  Contractor
    Eichberg Construction
    Rockville, Maryland

  Photographer
    Andy Lautman
    Washington, D.C.

ARCHITECT'S STATEMENT

This clinic provides maternal and child care for uninsured, low-income Hispanic families. Everyone working here is bilingual. Extensive social services and education are provided in conjunction with health care.

When Mary's Center outgrew its rented basement space, several grants allowed the organization to find a building to buy and renovate. Despite budget limitations, the center's goal was to create a striking and cheery place. Research revealed that children feel good in boldly patterned environments. This was used as a guide in designing the finished surfaces of this child-oriented place. The design team worked extensively with the staff to create the design.

The existing building was actually composed of five small structures built at different times for different uses and with different structural systems. They all had different floor levels. The resulting building had been combined in a way that ensured all visitors were lost once they left the front door. Providing orientation for patients was a high priority in renovation plans.

Orientation was achieved by creating a strong central space and using colors to define the different functional areas. The pediatric circulation is a loop to avoid congestion. The education and patient-receiving rooms are prominent at the ends of axes. Some floors were lowered and ramps installed to create handicap access to all spaces. The interior was totally reconfigured while preserving the existing structural systems to save on construction costs.

The large number of young children in the clinic, combined with the dispersal of some counseling offices, created acoustical problems. These were solved in part by providing a glass-enclosed play area for children in the waiting area and by heavy insulation and weather stripping at counseling room doors.

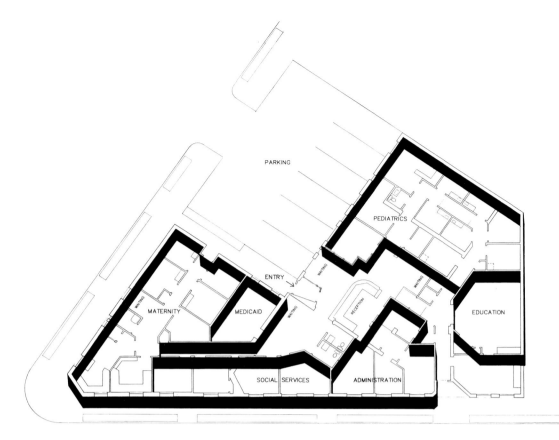

FUNCTIONAL ORGANIZATION

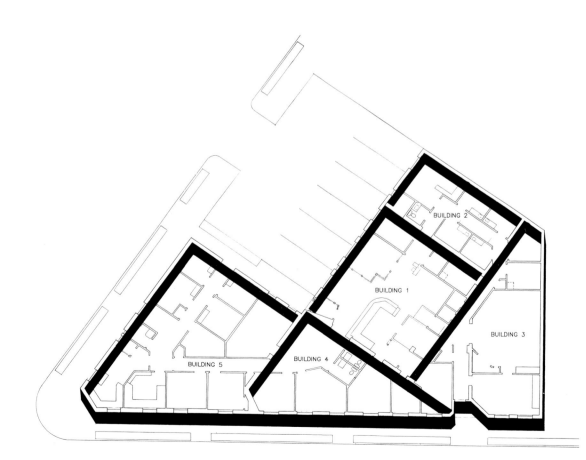

EXISTING BUILDING STRUCTURE

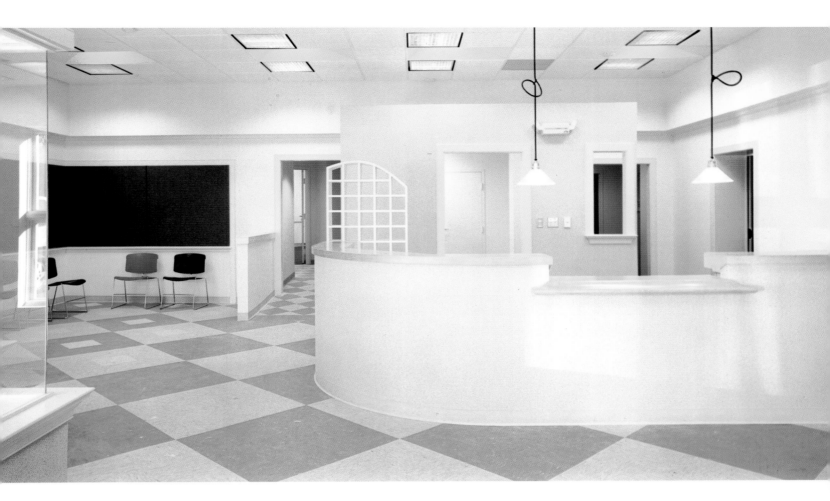

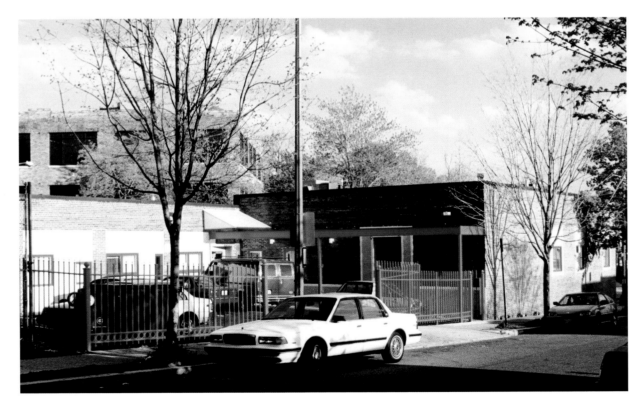

Centro Medico de la Mujer, Hospital Los Angeles

Torreon, Coahuila, Mexico

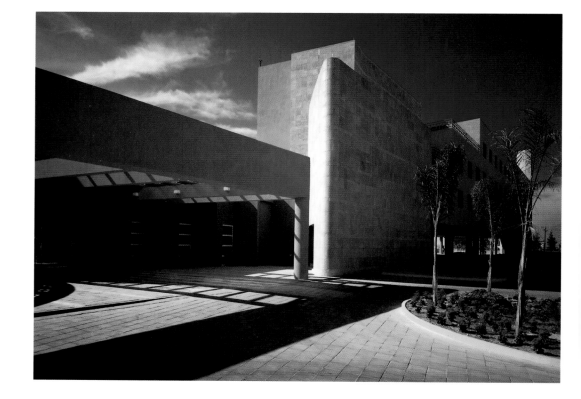

Owner
ABA/Inmuebles S.A. De C.V.

Data

Type of Facility
Women's hospital

Context
Freestanding

Type of Construction
New

Area of Building
68,837 GSF

Cost of Construction
$10,438,822

Medical Equipment Costs
$1,588,695

Status of Project
Completed December 1994

Credits

Architect
Henningson, Durham &
Richardson, Inc.
12700 Hillcrest Road, Suite 125
Dallas, Texas 75230-2096

Associate Architect
Fernando Siller Rodriguez
Arquitectos
Boulevard Independencia, 121 Ote.
Torreon, 2030 Coahuila, Mexico

Structural Engineer
Analysis Y Proyextos Racionales
S.A.
Torreon, Mexico

Mechanical/Electrical Engineer
Henningson, Durham &
Richardson, Inc.
Dallas, Texas

*Medical Equipment Planning
Consultant*
Mitchell International
Skokie, Illinois

Kitchen Consultant
Systems Design International
Dallas, Texas

Financial Consultant
ABA/Salud
Torreon, Mexico

ARCHITECT'S STATEMENT

The challenge in programming and designing this 30-bed women's hospital and medical office building was to blend attributes of Mexican culture with the latest in medical technology. Courtyards, gentle flowing curves, and peaceful colors are positive features within this health care environment. The geometric division of the site and massing of the building centers around a diagonal line, visually extending the main access road from its surroundings through the site. Serving a population of approximately 2.5 million, the hospital includes parking for 240 cars and a three-story medical-office building housing 50 physicians. The entire first floor of the facility is dedicated to the hospital.

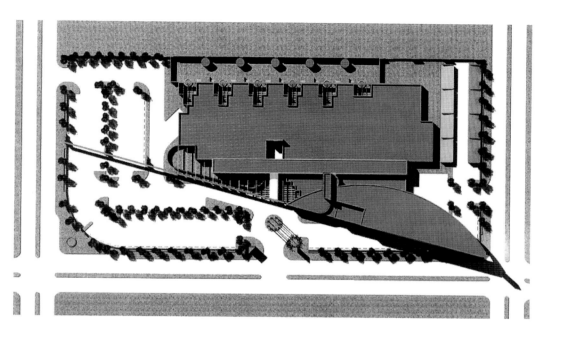

Credits (continued)

Contractor

Plate
Garza Garcia, Mexico

Photographer

Mark Trew, Studio 3i
Dallas, Texas

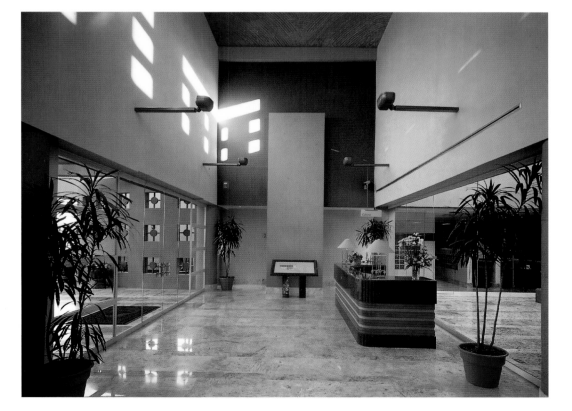

Deaconess Hospital OB/LDRP Renovation

Cleveland, Ohio

Owner
Primary Health Systems, L.P.

Data

Type of Facility
Women's hospital

Context
Hospital-based: 13 beds,
16 nursery beds

Type of construction
Renovation

Area of Building
12,600 GSF

Cost of Construction
$1,200,000

Medical Equipment Costs
$300,000

Status of project
Completed October 1994

Credits

Architect
HFP/Ambuske Architects, Inc.
21403 Chagrin Boulevard
Cleveland, Ohio 44122

Mechanical/Electrical Engineer
Bacik Karpinski Associates, Inc.
Cleveland, Ohio

Interior Design
Triad Design
Cleveland, Ohio

Contractor
Bolton Pratt Company
Cleveland, Ohio

Photographer
Trepal Photography, Inc.

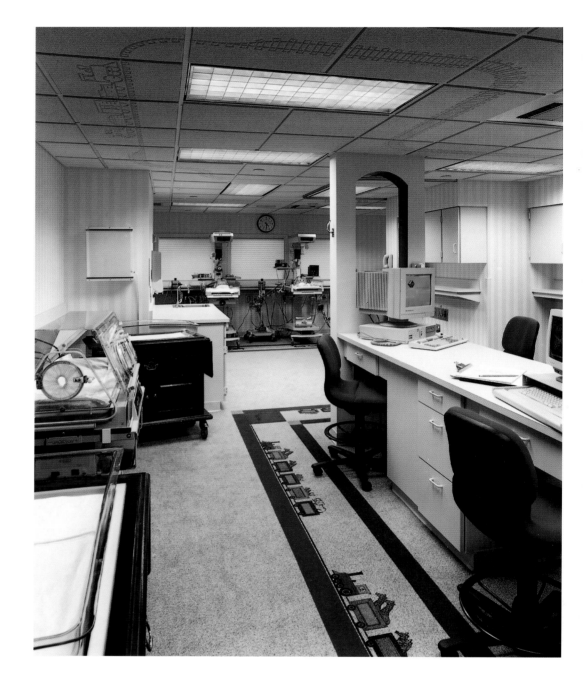

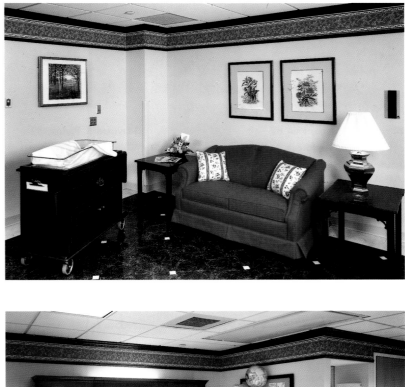

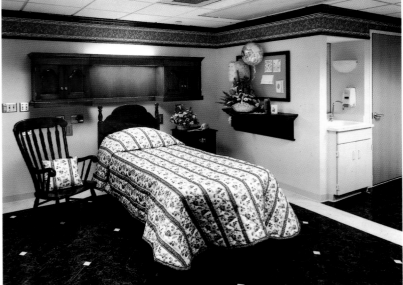

A R C H I T E C T ' S   S T A T E M E N T

This LDRP renovation program was converted through a five-phase construction project, changing a 20-year-old traditional program to a patient-focused women's center concept. The existing program included 23 beds, four labor rooms, one birthing room, two delivery rooms, and a 28-bassinet nursery. The new program includes seven labor/delivery/recovery rooms, three semiprivate postpartum rooms, one cesarean-section room, and a 16-bassinet nursery. The renovated unit has a residential environment and features upgraded mechanical/electrical systems and remodeled support space to improve staff efficiency.

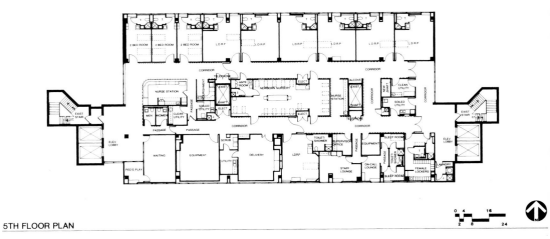

5TH FLOOR PLAN